HAVING
EPILEPSY

HAVING
EPILEPSY

The Experience and Control of Illness

Joseph W. Schneider
and
Peter Conrad

Temple University Press
Philadelphia

1/1984
Soc.

Temple University Press, Philadelphia 19122
© 1983 by Temple University. All rights reserved
Published 1983
Printed in the United States of America

Library of Congress Cataloging in Publication Data

Schneider, Joseph W., 1943–
  Having epilepsy.

  Bibliography: p.
  Includes index.
  1. Epilepsy—Social aspects. I. Conrad, Peter,
1945–   II. Title. [DNLM: 1. Epilepsy. WL 395
S359h]
RC372.S29   1983   362.1'96853   83-9153
ISBN 0-87722-318-1

To our fathers
C. William Schneider and George Conrad

Contents

viii

Contents

Preface

This book explores what it is like to have epilepsy and how people experience and attempt to control chronic illness in their everyday lives. Our respondents' words—the many quotes from the interviews we conducted—address the first theme most directly. The way we as sociologists have organized these quotes into the chapters that make up the larger book reflects the second theme. Thus, we believe the book speaks to several audiences (in no special order): to people with epilepsy and with other chronic illnesses; to their family members and friends; to various helping professionals whose work brings them in contact with those who have epilepsy, and to sociologists and other social scientists interested in the study of health and illness.

Although many social scientific studies examine various aspects of patienthood, being a patient of a doctor or being in a hospital represents only a small part of the total

xii
HAVING EPILEPSY

experience of having a chronic illness. Our study examines some of these everyday aspects of illness experience. This means that while we do consider physicians and professional medical care, we do not assume that the medical perspective is the only, or even the most insightful, way in which to understand illness experience. In fact, a medical point of view tends to minimize or ignore most of what we give central importance to here.

While illness does sometimes devastate people's lives, it also provides an opportunity to observe and appreciate the social processes of struggle, adaptation, and even success at gaining a sense of control over life's difficulties. We believe that this is an optimistic side of illness that is rarely considered. We came away from many interviews with a new respect for the human capacity to survive and get on with life, sometimes against great social and personal odds. Our respondents' stories seem best summarized by the experience of being assaulted followed by the struggle to regain a sense of control and order in their lives.

There are people and organizations to thank for their support, encouragement, and assistance in this project. Above all, we are grateful to the eighty people who agreed to share part of their lives with us. Without them this book would not exist. One person with epilepsy deserves special mention. Rita Dohrmann was a friend and early collaborator on this project. She was a sociologist and her insights about relevant questions and particular meanings were most valuable. Rita died tragically soon after the research began. We received vital financial support for interviewing and clerical help first from the Drake University Research Council, and later, from the National Institute of Mental Health Small Grants Section (MH 30818-01) and the Epilepsy Foundation of America. Portions of Chapter Seven have appeared in our paper, "In the closet with Illness: Epilepsy, stigma potential and information control," *Social Problems* 28, no. 1 (October 1980): 32–44, and we are grateful for the opportunity to expand on them.

The critical comments of the following people helped us improve various drafts of parts of this book and, in several instances, to see more clearly what we were doing: Gary Albrecht, Libby Bradshaw, Andy Gordon, John Kitsuse, John McKnight, Anselm Strauss, Steve Whitman, and Irving Kenneth Zola. Deborah Byers and Laurel Ingram helped with the tedious job of transcribing interviews. Dee Malloy deserves particular appreciation for her assistance in transcribing interviews, keeping our grant accounts ordered, and ably handling all manner of other administrative work. Jean Rider provided important research and typing assistance toward the end of the project. We would like to thank Carol Kromminga and Claudia Frazer for creating the index. Michael Ames of Temple University Press helped us with his enthusiasm for our project at a time when it was needed, and Zachary Simpson did a superb job of editing the manuscript. Nancy Schneider and Libby Bradshaw, as always, gave us much appreciated support and love.

HAVING
EPILEPSY

ONE

The Sociology of Illness

Illness has been studied primarily as something to be explained, eradicated, and controlled, usually by doctors. Medical culture and personnel are *the* authority on what illness is and what are the important questions to ask about it. One consequence of this has been that distinctions between illness and disease have been blurred. While illness and disease are related, they are not the same. Disease is understood best as an undesirable physiological process or state. Illness, in contrast, has less to do with problems of body per se than with the social and psychological phenomena that accompany these putative physiological problems (Feinstein, 1967; Freidson, 1970).

Illness is a *social* phenomenon that may or may not

rest on disease as a foundation. To say that illness is social is to emphasize the common experiences, activities, feelings, insights, relationships, and problems that surround sickness in social life.

We take this to be the "sociological perspective" on illness. But, to date, the sociology of illness has consisted mainly of studies that (1) search for various "social factors" believed to be causally related to disease, such as occupation, gender, and life stress; (2) define illness solely as "sick role" or patient behavior; (3) detail how conceptions of illness vary cross-culturally, and (4) examine how and under what circumstances people perceive symptoms and seek medical care (for an overview of this work, see Estes and Gerard, 1979; Litman, 1976; Kendall and Reader, 1979). Conspicuous by their rarity are studies of the *experience of illness*, of what it is like to be sick in society. There is little systematic data, for example, on what it is like to be a person with diabetes, arthritis, heart disease, cancer, or epilepsy. In this book, we seek to present an analysis and to tell the story of what it is like to have epilepsy. Beyond that, we suggest how the experience of illness can be conceptualized and studied.

MEDICINE, SOCIOLOGY, AND ILLNESS: OUTSIDER PERSPECTIVES

Modern medicine is essentially a practical enterprise. Both in its routine practice and in the scientific research and technology that support it, medicine is organized around defining lay complaints as evidence (or, not as evidence) of medical problems and then applying various "solutions."* The physician who "understands" a complaint but who cannot offer effective treatment receives little

---

*The medical jurisdiction is large and expansive. As Irving Zola (1972: 495) has argued, "If anything can be shown . . . to affect the inner workings of the body and to a lesser extent the mind," then it is

public or colleagial praise. Sociology, by contrast, is not primarily a practical enterprise in that its mission as a social science is to describe and analyze patterned aspects of social life. Direct intervention by sociologists toward bringing about social change garners little if any prestige in the profession. On this criterion, then, medicine and sociology are distinct. Sociology is closer to being a "pure" or "basic" science; medicine is more "applied."

Medicine and sociology have been similar, however, in their approach to the study of illness; both have been characterized by "outsider" perspectives in that the important questions for study are those of etiology and effective treatment. While such questions are certainly worthy, they produce knowledge that tells only a part of the story of illness. They allow little if any attention to what it is like to be sick, that is, what illness "looks like" from *inside* the experience.

The predominance of this outsider's view has a well-established historical precedent. A similar perspective has dominated thought and writing on crime, delinquency, and deviance; in short, on morally problematic behavior. David Matza (1969) has called this the "correctional" approach. It is an instructive parallel to most medical and social science research and writing on illness.* Matza argues that the most important questions in the study of crime and deviance have been, in effect, "Why do they do it?" and "How can we make them stop?" Those studying illness have asked, for the most part, "What causes it?" and "How can we stop or control it?" These questions rest on the assumptions first, that the thing being studied is so odious, so undesirable that the only reasonable course of action is to seek its control, and second, that the best way to accomplish this is to search for its causes. This ordering is not arbitrary. The

---

likely to be deemed a medical problem and thus to require medical solutions.

*We have argued elsewhere (Conrad and Schneider, 1980) that this correctional parallel may be seen clearly in the history and process of the medicalization of deviance.

disapproval or defined undesirability of a condition or conduct is itself an impetus for the search for causes. For more
than a century this task has been considered primarily the
province of professional medicine. Aside from the progress
such questions have stimulated, and in the study and control of disease it has been considerable, their predominance has discouraged the asking of other questions about
illness—namely, about what it is like to be sick in a world
that is, or appears to be, well. In our rush to control disease
we have neglected the detailed contours of illness as a lived,
personal and social experience.

The professional and cultural dominance of a medical,
outsider's view of illness as disease (see Freidson, 1970)
has made it difficult for social scientists themselves to see
what a distinctly social conceptualization of illness would
include. Social scientists have often defined their own research questions in light of these dominant views of illness.
On balance, social science has contributed to and elaborated upon the medical view of illness. It has commonly
reproduced medical concerns. This is most clear in social
epidemiological studies, popular since the 1950s, of relationships between suspected causal "social factors" and
the incidence and prevalence of diseases. To understand
what causes disease, however, is to know little of how illness is experienced.

A distinctly sociological approach to illness, but one
still reflecting medical definitions, was pioneered by Talcott Parsons (1951) in his concept of the "sick role." Parsons described illness as social deviance that needs to be
controlled by the medical profession to insure personal
and social stability. Illness, if unchecked, threatens the stability of the social group and society by opting people out
of essential role performances, such as those of work and
family life. This deviance, Parsons argued, requires a control mechanism that mollifies the threat and reintegrates
the sick individual into society as "well" or, at minimum,

as conforming to routine role demands. The medical profession and, in particular, the private relationship between the doctor and patient is precisely such a control mechanism. Stability and reintegration are realized when the patient conforms to sick-role expectations, exercising two well-known "rights"—exemption from playing routine roles and excuse from responsibility or blame for the condition—and acknowledging his or her "duties"—wanting to "get well" and seeking competent professional (meaning medical) help toward that end.

Parsons' sick-role concept has stimulated much social scientific research and writing (Levine and Kozloff, 1978; Twaddle, 1981) and remains a popular way to understand illness (Segall, 1976). It defines as important for study the topics of conformity to sick-role expectations, maintaining and optimizing the physician-patient relationship, and the stabilizing social consequences of adopting and relinquishing the sick role. In consequence, we have studied illness primarily in these terms. As with the ideas of correction and cause, the sick-role concept is like a pair of glasses with lenses ground to allow sight of some things while obscuring others. Wearing these glasses, the sociologist remains an outsider to aspects of illness experience these lenses do not bring into focus.

Given the influence of Parsons' conceptualization, it is not surprising to find a number of sociological studies that treat illness experience as synonymous with patient experience. It is of course true that part of being ill often does include being a patient. Only a relatively small amount of time, however, is spent by most sick people in direct interaction with doctors and/or in hospitals. Even when patienthood is examined in these studies, it often focuses not on the viewpoint of the patient but rather on the staff's view of patients (e.g., Lorber, 1975). This research grows out of the sick-role conceptualization and reflects its origins in studies of the doctor-patient relationship and of patients' compliance (or lack of it) with medical regimens and advice. Illness here remains very much something patients have and doctors treat in formal settings.

Somewhat as a corollary to the study of medical practice and still reflecting dominant medical culture, sociologists in the 1960s began to concern themselves with what happens to people before they arrive at the doctor's office, that is, how pre-diagnosis "symptoms" are perceived and how people come to seek medical care. Such conduct has been called "illness behavior," and in an early formulation, David Mechanic (1962: 189) defined it to include "the ways in which given symptoms may be differentially perceived, evaluated, and acted (or not acted) upon by different kinds of persons . . . whether by reason of early experience with illness, differential training in respect to symptoms, or whatever."

The study of illness behavior moves us closer to a bona fide sociology of illness experience. It nevertheless stops short of taking such experience seriously, on its own terms. While the experience of illness typically does begin before one becomes a patient, and does include patients' perceptions of their medical treatment (Zola, 1973), this work typically frames the experience in terms of the perception of and reaction to "symptoms," social networks used in locating help (Freidson, 1960), and the decision to seek medical care (Stimson and Webb, 1975). The convention has been to describe such behavior, its social and cultural variations, and then to explain how it affects connecting with professional medicine. The illness experience is a peripheral concern. Illness behavior studies, including research on illness careers (Suchman, 1965a, 1965b), draw attention more to the patient vis à vis health provider and/ or institutional context than to how such providers and contexts are seen and experienced.

Important though these studies may be, they do not give prime attention to before-diagnosis feelings, experiences, ideas and conduct. Too often, these are "packaged" into familiar sociological concepts or simply ignored. It is assumed that all roads lead ultimately and properly to professional care. The result is a doctor-and-hospital-centered view of illness, making receipt (or lack) of medical care the center of attention. Illness behavior studies often use outsider concepts such as "health beliefs" or sick role, or construct other analytic categories that give short shrift to the experience of illness itself (e.g., Robinson, 1971).

On balance, then, the sociology of illness has overlooked illness experience because it has adopted various outsider, usually medical, perspectives on what illness is and how it should be studied. Social epidemiology mirrors the medical search for causes of disease. Sick-role research seems more concerned with the role than the sickness. Research on the doctor-patient relationship and illness as patienthood usually focuses attention on conformity to institutionalized expectations rather than on how such "institutions" appear to sick people. Illness behavior studies address a segment of illness experience, but only insofar as it contributes or is related to care-seeking behavior and medical diagnosis.

THE EXPERIENCE OF ILLNESS: TOWARD AN INSIDER'S PERSPECTIVE

A bona fide illness experience perspective must consider people's everyday lives lived *with* and *in spite of* illness. Relevant questions include how people first notice "something is wrong" and what it means to them, what kinds of lay theories and explanations they develop to make sense of such strange and frightening events, how they come to seek medical care and with what concerns and expectations, what impact discovering their diagnosis has for them, and how they cope with a medical label and managing medications. We must examine relationships with family members, friends, and work associates. We must consider how people contend with formal and informal disenfranchisements based on a diagnosis, what it is like to make routine visits to the doctor or hospital, how these medical personnel look to patients rather than vice versa, and what strategies people use simply to "get by" in their lives. A developed insider's view of illness would address the ways in which people feel their disease, disorder, or disability has changed them in their own and others' eyes. It would, finally, confront questions of illness, self perception, and self worth. While not exhaustive, these issues begin to define an insider's view. The concerns and perceptions of sick and disabled people must be taken seriously as the "natural world" for scientific description and analysis.

This view draws from the sociological perspectives of symbolic interactionism (Blumer, 1969) and phenomenology (Schutz, 1971). Relevant assumptions from these traditions define the "natural" social world as a complex of meanings created by people as they interact. Social analysts confront these complex and shifting meanings whenever they study social life. This theoretical and research approach (sometimes called "qualitative") seeks to preserve and accurately render these patterns of meaning. This requires paying close attention to what people say and, to a lesser extent, what they do. Qualitative researchers, however, like all scientists and critics, seek to "go beyond" these data to "make sociological sense" of what they observe. We strive, in short, to do more than describe. We want to give our data (what Alfred Schutz [1971] has called "first-order constructs") sociological meaning ("second-order constructs") that produces new understanding without distorting what our respondents said.*

To apply this view to illness as a lived experience means we must take sick people's words, feelings, knowledge, and

---

*We generally agree with Bittner's (1973) position that there can be no true "insider's" view in sociological research (save, of course, of sociology itself), only a sociological rendering of it.

actions just as seriously as the medical scientist treats data from the laboratory. In its most complete application, it would produce an inclusive view of illness as a "career" (cf. Hughes, 1958; Goffman, 1959; Becker, 1963) having important moral elements. It would focus on how people perceive and manage conditions called illness in our society *beyond* how they manage *symptoms* and *medical care*. To the greatest extent possible, it would integrate participant-observation research with depth interviewing, yielding systematically collected data from people suffering a broad range of illnesses in a variety of settings. It would include attention to the collective actions that surround illness, descriptions of the illness world, explanations of the culture of illness, and an analysis of how the ill interact with both the well and other ill people. It would examine the emotional texture of experience and relationships with family members, friends, and work associates. Sociological and social science research on these and similar questions is rare and there is neither conceptual integration nor a developing systematic body of knowledge.*

There have been a few studies by sociologists that come close to or actually demonstrate this perspective. This work has been an inspiration and guide in our study of epilepsy and in thinking about the sociology of illness experience. Although our study may differ in emphasis, it builds upon these important works. Mark Zborowski (1952, 1969) documented different perceptions and reactions to pain across Jewish, Italian, and "Old American" ethnic groups in New York City. He found that pain is influenced by how people define it, but his study is quite specific and touches only a small segment of illness experience. Erving Goffman (1961) presented a patient's-eye view of mental hospitalization in *Asylums*, and Daisy Tag-

---

* It is interesting that while a book accounting for sociologists' experience of illness was published several years ago (Davis and Horobin, 1977), there is little published sociological research on the experience of illness.

liacozzo and Hans Mauksch (1979) examined the patient's view of hospital experience. Julius Roth (1963) took advantage of being a patient in a tuberculosis hospital to write a book called *Timetables*, about life inside the hospital. While it provides insight into illness experience, its limitation, from our view, is that it emphasizes the institutional dimensions of illness, such as the doctor-patient relationship in the hospital, rather than the totality of the experience itself. Fred Davis (1963) studied how children with polio and their families managed the "crisis" of this disease. Davis's study, however, is done more from the view of the children's parents than the children themselves. Davis concentrated on discovery and diagnosis, particularly how parents and physicians interact and define these situations. Barney Glaser and Anselm Strauss (1965, 1967) studied dying in the hospital and portrayed this experience, at least in part, from the perspective of the patient. Much attention, however, is given to staff-patient interaction, emphasizing how staff members manage dying.

Several studies have examined aspects of the experience of illness. Zachary Gussow and George Tracey (1968) conducted depth interviews with over one hundred leprosy patients. They examined how people manage the stigma of leprosy without suffering mortal wounds to their identities as worthy individuals. Gussow and Tracey found their respondents developed their own ideologies and theories about the stigma of leprosy to shield their selves. Marcella Davis (1973), David Stewart and Thomas Sullivan (1982), and Charles Waddell (1982) adopt similar perspectives to study people with multiple sclerosis and cystic fibrosis. Bill Cowie (1976) followed cardiac patients from the time they first perceived symptoms through their experiences with a doctor and in the hospital. He shows how these people first search for alternative, "normal" explanations of what is happening and how, after being told they had a heart attack, they reconstruct past events to make such an event understandable. The "worlds" of children dying of leukemia is the topic of a book by Myra Bluebond-Langner (1978). She spent nineteen months as a participant observer in a pediatrics department of a large hospital. She analyzes how these children came to know they were dying and how they managed this knowledge with parents, staff, and other children. Most of these studies, however, have been more of patienthood than of illness experience. We need insight into illness experience as it occurs outside such institutions, in everyday life and relationships.

Strauss and Glaser (1975), in a book made up of studies of chronic illness done by their students, give us the only collection of studies of illness experience outside institutional settings. These studies illustrate the kinds of issues such a perspective must address: the "burden of rheumatoid arthritis" (Wiener, 1975); "ulcerative colitis: strategies for managing life" (Reif, 1975); "getting around with emphysema" (Fagerhaugh, 1975); and "childhood diabetes: the commonplace in living becomes uncommon" (Benoliel, 1975). Strauss and Glaser discuss preventing and managing medical crises, managing medical regimens, controlling symptoms, the reordering of time, managing the course of the illness, social isolation, normalizing symptoms, and changes in relationships within the family. Strauss and Glaser (1975: viii) turn attention to how people "manage to live as normal a life as possible in the face of . . . disease. So the emphasis is very much on the social and psychological aspects (not the medical) of *living with chronic illness*." They are concerned with the way in which such illness seems to affect what they call the "quality of life."

Other sociologists and social scientists have noted the dearth of insider studies and suggest some directions to take. Robert Dingwall (1976: 132), after leveling an incisive critique of positivist, medically-influenced studies of illness, calls for studying "ethnomedicine," which he defines as: "The studies of the theories of body structure and function that members of a particular collectivity use to make sense of their own subjective experience and their observation of others." This may include, for instance, "ethnoanatomy, ethnophysiology, ethnopharmacology and so on." Dingwall argues that such studies must address "a crucial practical problem": "What is happening to me . . .?" Angelo Alonzo (1979) urges us to expand our sociological perspective to study "everyday illness behavior" that is rarely seen by doctors. He highlights in particular how people contain various illness symptoms and concerns within their everyday responsibilities and activities. Horacio Fabrega, Jr. (1979: 566) suggests we develop an "ethnography of illness" that would provide a careful description of the "orientations, concerns, and activities of persons who are judged as being ill or who believe themselves to be ill." Ellen Idler (1979: 725) calls for an approach to illness that would focus on "the subjective social reality of health and illness, and indigenous lay health beliefs and practices." She argues these areas have been "closed off" by our reliance on professional medical perspectives and assumptions about illness. Finally, David Locker (1981) has examined how people make sense of body/mind problems within the context of their everyday, commonsense understandings of health and illness.

In short, the study of illness experience is undeveloped and only vaguely conceived. There are, of course, many insightful first-person as well as literary accounts of being sick, but they remain unconnected and are usually based on the experiences of one or two people. Most sociological studies, even when they adopt an insider's perspective on illness, focus more on the experience of going to the doctor, being a patient, and/or being in the hospital.* Studies of the experience of illness need to be grounded in systematically-collected, first-hand data, and analyzed

* A recent exception is Irving Kenneth Zola's (1982a) unique personal account of his experience as a disabled person and his visit to Het Dorp in the Netherlands.

within a sociological or social psychological framework. We intend this book to be such a contribution.

STUDYING EPILEPSY: DATA, SAMPLE, AND METHOD

Given our commitment to an insider's view of illness, the general question that guided our study of epilepsy is, "What is it like to have epilepsy in this society?" Our research procedures followed directly from this question. The answer could come only from people as they spoke openly and freely about their lives. We were not concerned with how others, including physicians and various "experts," might answer this question. Consequently, our data consist of the *perceptions* of the experience of epilepsy by people who have this condition (which, of course, also present a limited, one-among-others, picture of epilepsy). Strictly speaking, these data are phenomenological in that they are the mental constructions linked to people's experience rather than researcher-constructed records of the events or conversations described. For us, the important thing is the perception, which can be analyzed quite independently of the question, "what *really* happened?"

Such data have integrity in their own right. They allow a greater understanding of the experience; they open one window through which we may see illness. Moreover, it is likely that these perceptions are important resources people draw on to guide and inform their conduct. Our results can give those with epilepsy—as well as those who give service—new insight on both how they and others might live with and understand this experience.

Epilepsy is a particularly good case for studying the experience of illness. There is a long history of its changing definitions and meanings that affect illness experience. The stigma potential of epilepsy is considerable, which makes possible a specific analysis of the relation between stigma and illness. Some evidence suggests that the stigma is more difficult for people to manage than the disorder itself (Commission for the Control of Epilepsy and Its Consequences, 1978). Although epilepsy is stigmatized, except for seizures it has low visibility as an illness. Thus, people with epilepsy can appear to be (and by some definitions are) "in good health" and lead conventional lives. They must, nevertheless, continue to manage aspects of their illness. Seizures are "surprise events" that can occur at any moment, disrupting life and causing embarrassment. People develop strategies for managing seizures and protecting self and "face." Because people with epilepsy generally make regular contacts with medical providers, and must take medications daily, it also offers the opportunity to examine medical care in people's everyday lives. Finally, there already has been some sociological work on epilepsy (Bagley, 1971; West, 1979a, 1979b; Oliver, 1980).

For this study we interviewed eighty people with epilepsy. These interviews ranged over a three-year period from 1976 through 1979 and lasted between one and three hours. They were guided by roughly fifty open-ended questions [see Appendix] covering various facets of people's lives. The interviews were tape recorded and yielded over 2,000 single-spaced typed pages of transcribed material. Respondents ranged in age from fourteen to fifty-four years (average age twenty-eight); we interviewed forty-four women and thirty-six men. Most came from a metropolitan area in the midwest. One of us interviewed a small number of people from a major city on the East coast. Our sample could be described as middle to lower-middle class in terms of education and income [see Appendix for more detail]. None of our respondents were or had been institutionalized in any long-term care facilities as a result of their epilepsy; none were interviewed in hospitals, clinics, or physicians' offices. In short, our sample and study were independent of medical and institutional settings. This is, as we noted above, unusual for research on illness. Most studies, even those that attempt to present an experience-of-illness viewpoint, have been done in or in conjunction with hospitalization or institutionalized medical practice.*

The sample is based on availability and willingness to participate. The option of drawing a statistically random or representative sample of people with epilepsy is precluded by the associated stigma and the lack of any reliable listing of people with this condition (something that is partly a product of this stigma). Even if such a sample could be drawn, the technical advantage of being able to draw statistical inferences to the larger population of people with epilepsy is of little interest to us. We were concerned instead to discover the contours of epilepsy as a lived experience: of how people deal with epilepsy and make sense of it as a part of themselves. We hoped to learn more about such experience and to gain insight into the general process through which people contend with illness. We were less interested to count the relative frequency of this or that kind of *person* with epilepsy than to begin to develop a clearer sense of the range of experiences that define the *world* of people with this condition. This dictated a "grounded theory" approach (Glaser and Strauss, 1967; Glaser, 1978) in which we sampled life situations, kinds of experiences, and ways of coping rather than personal attributes. Such "theoretical sampling" means that knowledge and insights gained in early interviews inform the choice of topics and situations to be discussed in later interviews.

We chose our sample by what is called the "snowball" technique, meaning we relied on word-of-mouth communication about our research from those interviewed to other people with epilepsy, on newspaper advertisements, on announcements of our project posted in local public

---

*Since most people with illness are not institutionalized, and only a small part of being ill involves being a patient, it is important to study ill people in nonclinical, noninstitutional settings, such as at home, in their leisure time, and at work.

areas, on assistance of various rehabilitation counseling agencies, on epilepsy self-help groups, on some medical personnel, and on letters from us to anonymous potential respondents passed by friends who had mentioned that they knew someone with epilepsy. We cannot, then, presume to know how much or how little our sample is like the larger category of "people who have epilepsy."

We analyzed our data using qualitative procedures that emphasize the search for and use of emergent "themes" (see Glaser and Strauss, 1967; Glaser, 1978; Lofland, 1971). This strategy combines data and analysis, rather than having analysis begin after all data are created. Early in our study we drew on the insight and experience of a colleague (an early collaborator) who herself had epilepsy. In addition, we conducted roughly fifteen pilot interviews that provided us with new areas of concern and new questions. We focused attention on recurrent themes and experiences as we conducted more interviews, eliminating some questions or giving them less attention. We read each other's transcripts from the first interviews to the last, offering suggestions for how to improve questioning strategy, style, and content.

In our coding, we attempted to preserve as much information as possible, while at the same time drawing out common features of the data. Rather than coding and classifying persons, we coded our respondents' perceptions and reported experience. We did this coding by using categories made up of words people used to talk about their concrete experiences. In addition, we developed codes based on more abstract, sociologically relevant concepts. As we did this coding, we wrote memoranda to ourselves and each other seeking to connect the concrete codes with the more abstract categories of sociological interpretation. For example, we wrote several memos on respondents' anguish and frustration about not being able to drive (the concrete code) as an example of others' reactions to putatively "dis-abled" people (the more general category). Other concrete coding categories include "seizures," "jobs," "family," and "medication." More abstract codes to which these concrete experiential categories were linked are "threats to self," "competence," "stigma," "information control," "lay theories," and so on. The results of such coding are, of course, reflected in the themes of our chapters.

OUTLINE OF THE BOOK

Now that we have given something of the context and direction of our study of epilepsy and illness, we can describe how the balance of the book is organized. Chapter Two, "The Historical and Social Realities of Epilepsy," examines the origins and major definitions of this condition, from ancient times to the present. A good deal of the experience of epilepsy comes from people confronting "what it is," meaning what it has come to be as a social object and the kinds of practices, both formal and informal, that surround it. Chapter Three, "Discovery," describes our respondents' first realizations that "something is wrong," their subsequent contact with physicians, and the nature and impact of learning their diagnosis. Chapter Four, "The Other Side of Care: Parents and Family Life," attempts to examine parents and family members through our respondents' eyes, particularly how they helped make sense of epilepsy and how it should be handled. Chapters Five and Six address the important topic of seizures, first, as assaults on self and self-control, and then as grounds for various strategies people develop and use to regain some of this threatened control. The stigma of epilepsy is the topic of Chapter Seven, "The Problem of Stigma: Managing Information." One of the dilemmas people with epilepsy (and perhaps other illnesses) face is whether or not to tell others, whom to tell, why, and under what circumstances. Chapter Eight, "Ties That Bind and Free: The Paradox of Medical Care," raises the paradox of respondents' relationships with doctors. Chapter Nine, "The Meaning of Medications," explores how people gain a sense of control by managing their own medication practice. In the the closing chapter, "Having Epilepsy: The Experience and Control of Illness," we attempt to draw the insights from our study of epilepsy together with relevant results from other research to suggest an agenda for studying illness experience. For those interested, an appendix on strategies and problems we encountered in this research follows.

TWO

The Historical
and Social Realities
of Epilepsy

Illnesses have historical and social realities that may be studied independently of how people experience them. In fact, to understand the experience of illness, we need to know more about what diseases and illnesses are as social objects, meaning as things on which people base their thought and action. What a disease or illness is in this social sense is not determined by any biophysiological process, nor is it obvious. The definition, meaning, treatment of, and response to an illness vary by social, cultural and historical context. The social reality affects how people experience illness as well as how others treat them. This is true for illnesses as different as cancer (Sontag, 1978), hyperkinesis (Conrad, 1975) and hysteria (Veith, 1965). The social reality is simultaneously an

historical reality, with current meanings an
reflecting those of the past.

The social and historical realities surrour
make it a particularly fearful and confusing
suddenness of a seizure, with its attendant ╌ ╌ ╌ ╌ ╌ body
control and its bizarre movements, can be frightening to
any uninitiated witness. What is happening? Is the individual all right? Should I do anything? Will he or she harm me?
Loss of self control may in itself be considered deviant and
justification for questioning an individual's social competence. What does this loss of control mean? Beyond this fear
of the epileptic * and his or her loss of control, the witness
fears for the safety of the sufferer. Historically there has
been particular concern about the dangers of falling into
water or fire. Misunderstandings, such as the belief the individual might swallow his or her tongue, are widespread.
These ideas not only reinforce fear of the epileptic, but they
combine with the observer's fear to profoundly influence
the person's own experience of epilepsy. Between seizures
it is quite possible for people with epilepsy to lead conventional and noteworthy lives. But that possibility is lessened
by the nonbiomedical realities that ultimately can play such
a role in shaping their experience.

HISTORICAL NOTES

Epileptic seizures, taken as the foremost physical sign
of the condition, have not changed through the ages. What
has changed are the meanings attributed to them. The earliest available records tell us that even in antiquity epilepsy
was defined as a disease and was held in contempt. The
conceptions and treatments of epilepsy changed with the

---

* One of our contentions in this book is that for most people the
reality is that they have epilepsy rather than that they are "epileptic."
We use the term occasionally in this book because it is the common historical designation, but it is a word that tends to label a person rather
than to describe a condition.

waxing and waning of medical and social definitions. Social barriers were erected and then removed, only to be erected in another form. Medical misconceptions and half-truths abound in the history of epilepsy. Dr. Oliver Wendell Holmes said, "If I wished to show a student the difficulties of getting a truth from medical experience I would give them a history of epilepsy to read" (quoted in Lennox and Lennox, 1960: 12).

The word epilepsy comes from the Greek word meaning "to take hold of" or "to seize" (*Oxford English Dictionary*, 1933). This describes the essence of epilepsy. When someone is "seized" by a convulsion, he or she typically falls to the ground, displays contorted bodily movements, makes grunting noises, salivates uncontrollably and loses consciousness. To the uninitiated observer, an epileptic seizure can be a frightening event. The person appears to be out of control, exhibits bizarre movements, and is unable to communicate with others.* There is no immediately available explanation of these movements and sounds for the observer. It certainly appears as if the person has been "taken hold of" by some alien force. The nature of this supposed "force" behind seizures has shifted with the historical period, and interpretations reflect ideas and belief systems popular or dominant at the time. The Devil, "gods," supernatural spirits, unbalanced body humors, and, most recently, electrical disturbances in brain functioning, have been credited with causing seizures.

Epilepsy always has been considered a disease, at least by some.† *On the Sacred Disease*, attributed to Hippocrates and written in 400 B.C., argues forcefully that epilepsy is a physical disease and not a divine or sacred one. This work was an attack on another, probably then-dominant

---

*These are the most obvious and extreme forms of seizures. There are also different and less total forms of seizures, which we mention later.

†We relied very much on Temkin's (1971) history of epilepsy when writing this section.

notion that epilepsy is a "possession" by demonic or supernatural spirits. The presumed presence of God or demons during a seizure made it a "bad omen" for the community. This made their occurrence troublesome not just for those who witnessed them, but for all in the social group.

The general notion from antiquity through the Middle Ages was that disease was a retribution for sin. Uncontrolled seizures made epilepsy particularly fearful and repulsive, further alienating the epileptic from society. The magical conception of epilepsy as "the sacred disease" conceived of it as contagious and disgraceful, a contagion that could be avoided by "spitting back" at the epileptic. Magical cures such as drinking the blood of gladiators or treatment with human bones were common.

Medical definitions competed with the more popular supernatural ones. Aretaeus, the Greek physician, concluded that "epilepsy is an illness of various shapes and horrible" (quoted in Temkin, 1971: 36). According to Galen, the great Roman physician, an "attack might originate from the brain directly, or the brain might be affected either by the stomach or any other part of the body" (Temkin, 1971: 37). The Hippocratic physicians theorized that diseases were caused by natural forces, specifically an imbalance of the four body humors or fluids. Epilepsy was usually depicted as caused by an imbalance of blood and phelgm. Treatment for epilepsy, when given, consisted mostly of contemporary pharmacopia and dietary prescriptions. Inveterate cases were deemed incurable. Although medical definitions challenged supernatural conceptions of epilepsy, Temkin (1971: 9) concludes, "To the ancients the epileptic was an object of horror and disgust and not a saint or prophet as sometimes contended."

In the Middle Ages epilepsy was called "the falling sickness" or "the falling evil." All diseases were considered punishment for sin, but epilepsy was particularly singled out because of its association with possession. The victims were believed to be under the power of a supernatural being whose will dictated their conduct (Temkin, 1971: 86), and they were seen as tormented by evil spirits.

The principal rationale for the Western theological explanation of epilepsy resides in a biblical account of Jesus driving out the "unclean spirit" (St. Mark, IX, 14–29). A father brought to Jesus his son, who was stricken by attacks: "And whatsoever he taketh him, he teareth him; he foameth, and gnasheth with his teeth, and he pineth away" (quoted in Temkin, 1971: 91). After an attack Jesus "rebuked the foul spirit" and lifted the boy up. Neither Jesus nor the father called the boy epileptic, but they agreed the child had been possessed by an unclean spirit, which, in the end, was driven out.

The popular interpretation of this story is that the disease that called forth the unclean spirit was epilepsy. Temkin (1971: 96) suggests that "the Gospel itself, where Jesus was reported to have driven the demon out of the epileptic boy, makes the acceptance of a purely physical theory impossible." Thus, the story strengthened the popular connection between evil spirits, the Devil, and epilepsy. Dante illustrates this in *The Inferno*: "And as he who falls, and knows not how, / *By forces of demons to death drag him*" (quoted in Temkin, 1971: 98, emphasis added). The idea of contagion persisted, engendering a vague fear of contact with epileptics; there was a "dread of sinister power lurking behind the possessed and the epileptic" (Temkin, 1971: 115).

The dual belief systems of the Middle Ages, demonic possession and the medical view of epilepsy, coexisted. The Renaissance saw debates between these viewpoints, especially in the medical writings of Thomas Willis in England and Hermann Boerhaave in Holland. Willis argued that the central nervous system was the seat of epilepsy and Boerhaave contended that a precondition in the brain was necessary for the onset of epilepsy (Geist, 1962: 14). Notions of epileptic as prophet (including the doubtful legend of Mohammed's epilepsy) or genius (e.g. Julius Caesar or Alexander) did exist during this time but appear not to have been held widely. Epilepsy was considered an abominable disease. As Kent says to the despised Oswald in *King Lear*, "A plague on your epileptic visage" (quoted in Temkin, 1971: 164). Epilepsy not only had horrible symptoms, but also was widely believed to be incurable. Epileptics thus were pitied but held very much at arm's length.

By the end of the seventeenth century, two types of epilepsy were recognized: "idiopathic epilepsy originating in the brain itself and sympathetic epilepsy originating from some other organ" (Temkin, 1971: 202). A great many contradictory and unsatisfactory theories prospered over the following two centuries.

In the latter part of the Enlightenment epilepsy was considered increasingly a "natural" phenomenon. This shift was due more to a change in social beliefs that made witches and demons disappear (e.g., rationalization) than to medical progress. The changing social climate rather than scientific discoveries tilted the debate to the medical side. Medical theories of epilepsy were still speculative and influenced by the morality of the time. For instance, well into the nineteenth century medical literature depicted masturbation as one of the main causes of epilepsy (Temkin, 1971: 231). At the same time, however, as early as 1815, Esquirol distinguished two types of losing consciousness as grand mal and petit mal attacks. He defined grand mal as fully developed convulsions with a loss of consciousness, but the meaning of petit mal was left vague. Throughout most of the nineteenth century the distinction between epilepsy and hysteria was blurred.

The treatment of epileptics, however, changed in the nineteenth century. Epileptics came to be treated much like other social deviants and troublesome people; they were institutionalized in asylums (see Rothman, 1971). In the early part of that century they were frequently housed with the insane, furthering the popular connection between epilepsy and insanity. After 1850, special institutions for epileptics were built. In 1867 the "Epileptic and Paralytic Hospitals" in Blackwell's Island, New York, opened, and in 1891 the first separate institution at Gallipolis, Ohio, was established. The accumulation of cases in these "hospitals" contributed to the image of epilepsy as a distant and incurable disease. These institutions existed in some form well into the 1950s. In 1950 there were about 50,000 people with epilepsy in various types of institutions and psychiatric facilities (Commission for the Control of Epilepsy and Its Consequences, 1978: Vol. II, Pt. 1: 789).

Other ideas about epilepsy appeared in writing about psychiatry and criminology during the nineteenth century. Psychiatrists wrote about "epileptic furor" and "epileptic mania," both depicted as harboring great potential for violence. Dangerous epileptics had to be "officially" certified, usually by asylum physicians (Temkin, 1971: 269). Cesare Lombroso, the founder of positivist criminology, developed "scientific" notions of epilepsy as a cause for crime and violence. Dostoevski's characters illustrate the social ambivalence toward epilepsy: Smerdyakov in *The Brothers Karamazov* is a murderer with "bad heredity," while Prince Myshkin in *The Idiot* is a saintly character.*

In short, by the middle of the nineteenth century epilepsy was considered a "natural" disease, but one that produced potentially dangerous and deviant people who, in some cases, must be institutionalized.

Most scholars mark a change in the medical view of epilepsy with the work of John Hughlings Jackson (Temkin, 1971; Lennox and Lennox, 1960). Jackson was an esteemed and brilliant British neurologist who, beginning in 1862 and

---

*It is well known that Dostoevski had epilepsy. Most histories of the disorder list famous individuals who are believed to have suffered from epilepsy. Included are such luminaries as Julius Caesar, Alexander the Great, Caligula, Peter the Great, Socrates, Frederick Handel, Alfred Nobel, and Tchiakovsky. Some lists include others whose diagnosis is less certain, such as St. Paul, Mohammed, and Napoleon.

for the next forty years, published a variety of papers that laid the groundwork for the modern conception of epilepsy and profoundly influenced all of neurological science.

Jackson was a clinician who based his work on detailed observation of thousands of cases. His research in epilepsy stemmed from his more general interest in how "a symptom could reveal normal function and illuminate the normal dynamic properties of the nervous system" (Clarke, 1973: 47). His major work was identifying the unilateral or localized seizures, which are now called Jacksonian. "At a physiological level he considered a convulsion to be a symptom, not a disease per se: 'an occasional, an excessive and a disorderly discharge of nerve tissue on muscle'" (Clarke, 1973: 48). Jackson's idea of "discharge" anticipated and influenced the contemporary notion of seizures as electrical discharges. In his study of the underlying mechanisms of epilepsy (including the "psychomotor" and "temporal lobe" variants) Jackson provided the scientific foundation for understanding epilepsy as a biophysiological phenomenon. Temkin (1971: 381) concludes: "Jackson's great acheivement was the aligning of the epilepsies with modern physiology of the human nervous system, based on discharges of ganglionic cells and the co-ordination of human behavior with an evolutionary anatomy of the brain and spinal cord."

Jackson was not interested in the social aspects or moral evaluation of epilepsy; he was not concerned about whether the behavior was ridiculous, pathetic, or even criminal (Temkin, 1971). In a sense, Jackson's work represents a purely biomedical approach to epilepsy, seeing it only on a physiological plane. While this freed the medical and professional conceptions from many of their moralistic biases, it also ignored much of what having epilepsy means.

The first effective pharmacological treatments for epilepsy were introduced in the nineteenth century. Bromides, introduced in 1857, reduced the frequency and severity of seizures. Unfortunately, they also made people sluggish and disoriented. Drugs introduced in the twentieth century were both more effective and less troublesome: Phenobarbital in 1912, Dilantin (phenytoin sodium) in 1938, Mysoline (primidone) in 1952, and Sodium Valproate in the 1970s. These drugs controlled or minimized seizures for many people. The use of the electroencephalogram (EEG) in the 1930s allowed measurement of distortions of electrical activity in the brain and enabled a more specific and clear diagnosis. It is plausible to suggest that better diagnosis and anticonvulsant medications led to a reduction in discrimination against people with epilepsy by the 1950s. This could be due at least in part to the definition of epilepsy as a disorder that could be controlled medically.

Today, epilepsy is nearly completely medicalized. It is a medical disorder to be treated by medical intervention. The social aspects of epilepsy have been, in comparison, ignored and unstudied. But the history of epilepsy is a history of stigma. The social residues of these negative and pejorative conceptions remain alive as issues with which people having epilepsy must contend. In fact, as the Commission for the Control of Epilepsy and its Consequences (hereafter called the Commission Report) stated (1978: Vol. 1: 75): "Possibly the least understood and most neglected aspects of epilepsy are the social, psychological and behavioral problems that are so common." In the next section we explore and challenge some of the popular "myths" about epilepsy.

THREE MYTHS ABOUT EPILEPSY

Misinformation and mythology about epilepsy abound. The Commission Report attempted to clarify several common misunderstandings. For instance, epilepsy is not a disease. It is a symptom of a disorder in the brain. Epilepsy has no single "cause." It can affect anyone, at any age, and at any time. Epilepsy has many forms, ranging from violent convulsions to momentary lapses of attention. It is an episodic disability. Seizures usually are brief and infrequent, and between them, most people with epilepsy are perfectly normal and healthy. For most who have it, epilepsy can be treated, thus permitting many individuals to lead normal lives. All of this aside, epilepsy can carry with it a host of psychological and social problems. *"For many, it is not the disorder, but society's reaction to it that creates the disability"* (Commission Report, 1978, Vol. 1: 133; emphasis added).

A number of specific myths about epilepsy have emerged over the last century. We discuss three myths that are among the most pervasive and detrimental to people with this condition. These myths are particularly problematic because they each have received some degree of professional legitimation. That is, these ideas are sometimes reinforced by various professional people, perhaps most consequentially by physicians, who deal with epilepsy. These myths are, of course, prevalent among lay people as well. It is difficult to determine, historically, whether these myths emerged as professional/scientific versions of popular negative conceptions or whether professionals helped create such negative ideas. Most likely, there has been an interaction of these influences, but surely these myths have served to perpetuate and even legitimate epilepsy as a stigmatized disorder. These beliefs are myths not because they are totally invalid (although they may be) but because they are traditional and historical beliefs that at various times have been elevated to represent the "truth" about epilepsy and epileptics. As "truth" they are myths; stories from the past that still affect the experience of epilepsy.*

---

*We do not claim to exhaustively and definitively refute these myths—others have previously done this—but rather to point out some of their origins, content, and evidence.

MYTH 1: EPILEPSY IS AN
INHERITED DISEASE

This myth has two parts: first, that epilepsy is a disease; second, that it is inherited. The Commission Report pointed out that epilepsy—there defined as a seizure disorder—is better conceptualized as a symptom than a disease. Seizures are seen to be symptomatic of a variety of biophysical conditions and events. It is not a singular disease or even one disorder. Many physicians today speak of "the epilepsies," or avoid the term epilepsy altogether for "convulsive disorder" (which creates its own confusion).

The idea that epilepsy is inherited has a long history. Hippocrates argued, in *On the Sacred Disease*, that epilepsy, like all diseases, was hereditary. In the middle of the seventeenth century, Boerhaave contended that heredity was one of the most important factors causing a congenital predisposition to epilepsy (Geist, 1962: 14). In 1881, Gowers suggested that 30 percent of the cases of epilepsy was inherited, a high figure for any disorder (Temkin, 1971: 348). William G. Lennox, a distinguished expert on epilepsy, demonstrated that epilepsy was five times more frequent in relatives of epileptic patients than in the general population, and estimated that at least 35 percent of the cases was genetic (Lennox and Lennox, 1960). He argued for a congenital predisposition to seizure disorders rather than a direct inheritance of epilepsy.

Although the data are not available to definitively settle the question of the heritability of epilepsy, we can clarify some of the issues. In terms of cause, there are two major classifications for epilepsy. *Acquired* or symptomatic epilepsy is caused by detectable cerebral changes or damage (most commonly head trauma). *Idiopathic* or essential epilepsy means that the cause of seizures cannot be determined, and no cerebral or other lesion can be found. When we discuss heredity, we are only including idiopathic epilepsy and it is unclear how much of this category is genetic.

Recent reviews of the genetics of epilepsy argue that much of the evidence is contradictory (Bagley, 1971: 102–107; Newmark and Penry, 1980). Although the genetic transmission of epilepsy is unclear, it seems evident that in some but not all cases of idiopathic epilepsy a genetic factor is involved. For example, there is considerable evidence for hereditary patterns for epilepsy associated with the spike wave EEG trait (Commission Report, 1978, Vol. II, Pt. 1: 203). In a study of over 500 patients, Hauser and Kurland (1975) found that only 23.3 percent had known causes; 3.9 percent were classified congenital. Rodin (1978) found 8 percent likely or definitely hereditary, with another 15 percent possible. Newmark and Penry (1980: 95) estimate up to 10 percent of the children of epileptic parents (higher among affected mothers) have epilepsy. Overall, the data show that while there is no single genetic cause of epilepsy, there are numerous genetic factors involved, and probably many inherited diseases having seizures as a symptom (Commission Report, 1978, Vol. II, Pt. 1: 117). The Commission Report (1978, Vol. I: 30) concluded: *"Inheritance plays a very minor role in epilepsy despite the widely held misconception that epilepsy is inherited"* (emphasis added).

The myth that epilepsy is an hereditary affliction has contributed to a number of social policies adversely affecting people with epilepsy. Many restrictive laws and regulations have been based on the belief that epilepsy is an inherited disease. A 1757 Swedish law, in effect for over 150 years, forbade epileptics to marry (Newmark and Penry, 1980: 1). In 1895, Connecticut was the first state to pass a "eugenic marriage" law prohibiting marriage by persons with epilepsy. As late as 1952 seventeen states prohibited the marriage of persons with epilepsy (Kittrie, 1971: 312), although today epilepsy per se is no longer grounds for prohibiting marriage (Hughes, 1975: 55). In 1907, Indiana introduced the first "eugenic sterilization" law, aimed at preventing certain people with epilepsy (usually institutionalized) from reproducing; as of 1971, nine states still had such laws (Kittrie, 1971: 318). Immigration laws also restricted people with epilepsy. Prior to 1965, people with epilepsy were among those excluded from immigrating to the United States (under Title 8, U.S. Code 1182). This policy was based on the unfounded fear that people with epilepsy (and presumably their offspring) would become public charges (Lennox and Lennox, 1960, Vol. 2: 986). Even as defunct social policies, these laws distorted the image of epilepsy and advanced the negative social response. They depicted the epileptic as a biological defective who could not be trusted to manage relationships, bear children, or earn a living.

The assumption that epilepsy is a hereditary illness, particularly when the evidence was inconclusive or limited—which is to say most of the time—led to a variety of official discriminatory policies. Moreover, it took an uncountable toll on the everyday relationships and self concepts of people with epilepsy.

MYTH 2: EPILEPSY CREATES PSYCHOPATHOLOGY AND LEADS TO MENTAL ILLNESS

This ancient and widely-held belief permeates the professional literature as well as popular conceptions. Its origins are traceable to Hippocrates, who first hypothesized that the brain was the seat of epilepsy. In this context, the myth is understandable, given the intimate connection between the brain and personality, self, mind, and intelligence. An 1822 book claimed there was no distinction between lunacy and epilepsy, as both were governed by the moon (Highmore, 1822). Well into the 1970s, introductory and abnormal psychology textbooks continued to include epilepsy in sections covering "mental disorders."

This myth has manifested itself in the belief that people with epilepsy are of subnormal intelligence, that they often develop a peculiar and unpleasant epileptic personality, and that their epilepsy leads to psychopathology and mental disorder. These are variations on the theme that epileptics are mentally different from normal people.

Epileptics as Mental Defectives. In the late nineteenth century writings on epilepsy it was widely accepted that the condition caused mental deterioration and that dementia was a consequence of seizures. For example, Gowers wrote in 1881: "The mental state of epileptics . . . as is well known, frequently presents deterioration. . . . In its lighter forms there is merely defective memory. . . . In more severe degrees there is greater imperfection of intellectual power, weakened capacity for attention and often defective moral control" (quoted in Guerrant et al., 1962: 3–4). The term "epileptic dementia" occurs frequently in the psychiatric literature. For example, in 1899 two psychiatrists wrote, "The rate of progress of epileptic dementia is in direct proportion to the number and severity of seizures" (quoted in Guerrant et al., 1962: 4). No doubt this view was reinforced by clinical observation and study of institutionalized epileptics, where the effects of disorder and institutionalization cannot be separated (see Goffman, 1961). There is some evidence that the bromides then used to control seizures actually produced mental sluggishness (Hughes, 1975: 20).

With the advent of intelligence testing in the early twentieth century, researchers set out to "prove" that epileptics generally had subnormal intelligence. At least fifty-two studies were published in a twenty-year period connecting epilepsy to low mentality. By the 1950s, new studies were being published that refuted these earlier studies and argued that people with epilepsy have never differed significantly from the general population (Hughes 1975: 22). The intellectual function of people with epilepsy who have had no brain damage is similar to that in nonepileptic populations. A recent review of this research concludes: "In general terms there is no *good evidence*, in properly matched groups, *that there is any lowering of intelligence due to epilepsy itself*, although of course any causative brain damage may lead to intellectual loss and cognitive impairment" (Laidlaw and Richens, 1976: 151, emphasis added). The fact that a significant number of mentally retarded individuals also have epilepsy has perhaps also perpetuated the public image linking epilepsy and mental subnormality. There is no sound evidence that epilepsy causes mental retardation.

The Epileptic Personality. The notion that people with epilepsy have or develop a specific type of personality (usually antisocial in nature) has taken several forms. The Greeks believed that if epilepsy became chronic, the whole personality would be affected. Aretaeus wrote that epileptics became "languid, spiritless, stupid, inhuman, unsociable and not disposed to hold intercourse, nor to be sociable, at any period of their life" (quoted in Temkin, 1971: 44). Esquirol in his 1813 study found that no less than four-fifths of the women in his study were mentally affected. The term "epileptic personality" was coined by the nineteenth century French psychiatrist Moral (Temkin, 1971: 365). The late nineteenth century medical literature is replete with descriptions of epileptic deterioration and personality change. It was not, however, until the first few decades of the twentieth century that scientific research on the epileptic character appeared (Guerrant et al., 1962: 7–10). The neurologist L. Pierce Clark was one of the foremost and most influential proponents of the idea of the epileptic character. In 1917 he described the nature and pathogenesis of epilepsy:

> First, that there is invariably present an epileptic constitution or make-up in those individuals who later develop essential [that is, idiopathic] epilepsy. The nucleus of this personality defect is a temperament of extreme hypersensitiveness and egotism and all that these two main characteristics entail. This defect in character is not to be taken in any narrow or moralis-

tic sense, but is to be considered as a temperamental defect in a broad, biologic view, a personality-defect which makes its possessor incapable of social adaptation in its best setting and which, if it remains uncorrected, renders the individual entirely inadequate to make a normal adult life (Clark, 1917: 2).

In Clark's later writing (e.g. 1925: 28) and in the works of others we see the epileptic personality described repeatedly with such pejorative terms as irritability, supersensitiveness, antisocial, egocentric, disturbances of mood, impulsiveness, rigidity and consequent emotional poverty. By 1943 Grinker's textbook in neurology, while accepting and describing the epileptic personality in these terms, questioned whether these characteristics were essential to an epileptic character, or were, rather, a result of the "chronic invalidism of this tragic condition" (quoted in Guerrant et al., 1962: 12). Bagley argues that scientific studies, especially those before 1947, gave epilepsy a bad image. They were methodologically weak, used inadequate measurement and had no control groups. "A common feature of such studies was to associate epilepsy with a wide range of adverse traits, the evidence being either the authors' impressions of unspecified epileptic populations or the accretion of previous opinions" (Bagley, 1971: 26).

There is little research evidence supporting the notion of an antisocial epileptic personality. A study designed to test a variant of the epileptic personality hypothesis yielded negative results—that is, the epileptic group had no higher incidence of functional disorders than the controls with a variety of chronic illnesses (Guerrant et al., 1962). Today, to the extent that the idea of an "epileptic personality" survives in the medical literature, it is believed to be environmentally induced. A recent review concluded that a few patients under extreme conditions (e.g., institutionalization) "may develop a fairly characteristic pattern of personality change" (Laidlaw and Richens, 1976: 174). But where there are common characteristics, even among this small subgroup, it appears likely that they are a by-product of stress, stigma, discrimination, and socio-environmental conditions. There is literally no evidence to support the hypothesis of an inherent epileptic personality.

Epilepsy Leads to Psychopathology and Mental Disorder. It is just a short step from describing epileptic personality traits in disparaging terms to concluding that epilepsy leads to psychopathology and psychiatric disturbance. Between 1947 and 1966 several studies found the prevalence of "personality disorders" among people with epilepsy, ranging from 12 to 59 percent of those studied (Bagley, 1971: 46). After noting that the studies were methodologically poor and often contradictory, Bagley (1971: 47) concluded, "There seems to be general agreement, however, that personality disorders are much more common than in the general population." Bagley (1971), in a well-controlled study, proposed the interaction of a complex pattern of social, personality, and organic factors to explain the development of psychiatric disturbance in children with epilepsy.

More recent hypotheses have suggested that only particular forms of epilepsy are associated with psychopathology. The most common connection made by researchers is between psychomotor or temporal lobe epilepsy and mental disorder. F. A. Gibbs published a series of papers beginning in the late 1940s claiming a high incidence of psychiatric disorders between seizures in persons with psychomotor epilepsy (Guerrant el al., 1962: 13). Others echo the hypothesis that psychomotor or temporal lobe epilepsy itself is a determinant of psychiatric disturbance and personality disorder. But these studies also have been criticized for being methodologically inadequate. Moreover, one study designed specifically to test the temporal lobe hypothesis produced negative findings (Guerrant et al., 1962). A recent study using the MMPI (Minnesota Multiphasic Personality Inventory), a popular and well-respected psychological test, found psychosis to be no more associated with temporal lobe epilepsy than with generalized seizures (Hermann et al., 1981). This same research group, in a larger study comparing epilepsy with other chronic disorders, concluded that "groups of people with epilepsy do not manifest more psychopathology than other chronic illness groups. However, when psychological dysfunction is present, it tends to be more severe in epilepsy groups" (Whitman et al., 1981). Other recent research efforts suggest that the majority of epileptic patients is mentally normal, but as with all cerebral dysfunction, there may be an increased prevalence of psychological disorders (Reynolds and Trimble, 1982).

In short, the evidence on this connection is mixed and continues to accumulate. Whether epilepsy causes increased psychopathology remains an open question. To the extent there is a higher incidence of mental and emotional problems among people with epilepsy, it is equally likely to be a product of the social reaction to epilepsy. No research to date has systematically studied this hypothesis.

The assumption, however, that epilepsy itself causes psychopathology is widespread and has certain consequences. It stigmatizes people with epilepsy by linking them to mental illness, and it becomes especially damaging when it is institutionalized in certain official documents. For example, the *Corpus Juris Secondum*, a definitive source for all aspects of legal cases, defines epilepsy as follows:

a chronic disease of the nervous system, attended by general brain deterioration; which is progressive and congenital; and likely to be transmitted by marriage and childbearing, and is considered incurable. . . . Epilepsy is not to be regarded as a form of insanity in the sense that the person afflicted with it can be said to be permanently insane, for there may be little or no mental abberration between the attacks; but epilepsy may cause insanity, and temporary insanity in some cases, follow[ing] the proxysms, varying in different instances from the slightest alienation to the most violent mania, the latter form of the affliction known as "epileptic fury," and while it lasts, it may be considered as a state of insanity, during which the patient is deprived of reason and judgment. The course of epilepsy is one of deterioration [32 *Corpus Juris Secondum*, 1954: 612; quoted in Hughes, 1975: 9].

When myths about heredity, progressive brain deterioration, and psychopathology become ensconced in a prestigious legal resource, they are elevated to working assumptions of lawyers and others dealing with epilepsy. The consequence is to perpetuate unsupported allegations and to amplify stigma and discrimination.

MYTH 3: EPILEPSY CAUSES AGGRESSION AND CRIME

The association of aggression and crime with epilepsy has been pervasive in criminological circles for over a century.* Although its popularity in professional circles has waned in recent years, one still finds it mentioned in criminology textbooks and the popular literature.

The linking of epilepsy to deviance is hardly surprising given epilepsy's historical connection with the Devil and demons. Abulgasim, circa 1000 A.D., linked epilepsy to crime, citing the biblical connection of seizures with visitations from the Devil (Temkin, 1971: 106). But it was Casare Lombroso's positivist criminological theories that cemented the association. Lombroso, an Italian military physician who was deeply influenced by Darwin, observed that a large number of criminal offenders had tattoos. Lombroso began to look for other stigmata and subsequently developed a theory of the "born criminal." He soon expanded his theory to include the "insane criminal," which included epileptics (the "epileptic criminal"). Lombroso accepted the popular notion that epilepsy was a degenera-

---

*We are grateful to Marcia Kemper for background research for this section.

tive disease and argued that both epileptics and criminals were atavistic types—that is, "evolutionary throwbacks" to a more primitive stage of human development. He described one class of criminals as epileptoids, holding "the epileptic criminal, the insane criminal and the born criminal as separate types all stemming from an epileptoid base" (Mannheim, 1960: 185).

Lombroso's work had an enormous impact on the field of criminology as well as on popular thinking about crime and especially criminals. Many of his followers, such as Enrico Ferri, were central figures in connecting criminal behavior to biological causes. Other prominent psychiatrists and physicians, such as Henry Maudsley and M. Gonzalez Echeverria. provided variation on the epilepsy and crime hypothesis. Echeverria, in his 1872 study of David Montgomery, "cited cases [from the available literature] where epileptics had asked to be forcefully prevented from criminal acts to which they were driven by an irresistible impulse" (Temkin, 1971: 361). A number of poorly conceived studies attempted to demonstrate the connection. While Charles Goring disproved Lombroso's "born criminal" thesis in his 1913 book, *The English Convict*, it was not until C. L. Anderson's 1936 study that the epilepsy and crime thesis was adequately refuted. Anderson (1936) found that there was no statistical difference in the prevalence of epilepsy between the general population and the prison population. Since then there have been reports that people with epilepsy tend to be somewhat less criminogenic than the general population (Foxe, 1948, cited in Bagley, 1971: 78). One small study suggests that some incarcerated delinquents may be mislabeled as epileptic (Oliver, 1980).

The myth of the relationship between epilepsy and crime appears in some criminology textbooks. A 1967 textbook suggests that epilepsy is one, albeit very small, cause of crime and estimates that one percent of all crimes are caused by epilepsy.

Central to the argument relating epilepsy and crime is

the proposition that epilepsy specifically causes aggression and violence. One possible source of this thesis is the unpredictable and "violent" movements and loss of control exhibited during seizures—most especially those so-called "automatisms" characteristic of some temporal lobe seizures. Fabret, writing in 1863, described people having such seizures: "They strike mechanically, without motivation, without interest, without knowing what they do or, at least, with a very vague consciousness of their actions" (quoted in Temkin, 1971: 321). The epileptic aggression thesis also reflects the epileptic personality myth, and is fueled by the psychoanalytic studies that contend people with epilepsy possess aggressive drives, the repression of which causes seizures (Bagley, 1971: 26). While there is some evidence that temporal lobe epilepsy may be associated with aggressive behaviors, research results are far from consistent (see Bagley, 1971: 69). Some have argued that epileptics could commit murder during a seizure. Others have claimed that neurosurgery is a "cure" (Mark and Ervin, 1970), but this "treatment" has been severely criticized (Chorover, 1973).

The Commission Report (1978, Vol. II, Pt. 1: 351) stated that aggression is usually limited to a small portion of persons with temporal lobe epilepsy and it is "an uncommon extreme episodic irritability" rather than a product of this form of epilepsy. Recent research has added further doubt to the epilepsy-aggression connection. One study, comparing those with temporal lobe epilepsy and other people with epilepsy, found no support for the hypothesis that increased aggressiveness is associated with temporal lobe epilepsy (Hermann et al., 1980). An even more impressive study, conducted by an international task force of epilepsy experts, selected nineteen patients (out of 5,400 with epilepsy) who were believed to exhibit aggressive behavior during seizures. Using very rigorous criteria, they found that only seven of the nineteen patients actually exhibited aggressive behavior during seizures.

After careful review and observation, this panel concluded it was nearly impossible for a person to commit murder (or similar acts) during a seizure: "[T]he acts of aggression [require] a series of consecutive and sustained movements that [are] organized toward a purpose. As such, they are contrary to the nature of epileptic automatisms" (Delgado-Escueta et al., 1981: 715).

One of the strangest ideas in the history of epilepsy is the concept "epileptic equivalents." A considerable literature exists postulating that positive spikes on an EEG (similar to some seen with epilepsy) in a patient who exhibits deviant behavior indicate a possible organic cause of deviance. Some doctors have considered the behavior an "epileptic equivalent" (usually postulated to originate in the temporal lobe), even when there are no clinical manifestations of epilepsy, i.e., no seizures (see Bagley, 1971: 71–77). A few have called it a "syndrome" (Gross and Wilson, 1964). One investigator's assertion (Bennett, 1965), without evidence, that "many horrible crimes are attributable to epilepsy" (even among those without seizures), is a startling example of how the negative definition of epilepsy is used to "explain" deviant behavior.

In sum, there is virtually no support for the claim that epilepsy causes crime, and only slight systematic evidence relating epilepsy to aggressive behavior. This myth is an example of the medicalization of deviance, the creation of medical definitions and theories for deviant behavior. Medicalizing deviance has consequences that range beyond our discussion here (see Conrad and Schneider, 1980), but epilepsy's stigmatized status and behavioral manifestations make it likely that the link between epilepsy and deviance will continue to be advanced.

Myths such as these have perpetuated and legitimated the stigmatization of epilepsy. Although they are inaccurate and burdensome for people with epilepsy, they are part of the social reality with which they must live. In the next section we discuss some of the more concrete manifestations of the institutionalized stigma and discrimination surrounding this condition.

THE SOCIAL RESPONSE TO EPILEPSY: A STIGMATIZED ILLNESS

The history of the social response to epilepsy is replete with the social barriers that limit people's ability to lead conventional lives. We have already mentioned various attempts to separate "epileptics" from the normal population through explicit stigmatization, incarceration, hospitalization, marriage and sterilization laws, immigration restrictions, theories of dangerousness, or depictions of them as unreliable personalities. People with epilepsy must cope with official as well as informal discrimination. For instance, until 1982 a history of epilepsy disqualified a person from United States military service (*National Spokesman*, March 1982). Official public policies have reinforced as well as reflected negative cultural definitions of epilepsy. In this section we review some contemporary examples of issues concerning discrimination toward people with epilepsy.

Prejudicial ideas and discriminatory behavior are often, but not always, related. Prejudice points to what people say they believe or think; discrimination directs our attention to what they do, namely, treat various kinds of people unequally. Social scientists have known for some time that what people say does not necessarily reflect what they do (see Deutscher, 1973). Nonetheless, it is plausible to suggest that prejudice, as preconceived judgments, affects behavior toward the object of such judgments—in this case, epilepsy and people known to have it.

Researchers using Gallup Poll data have studied the American public's attitude toward epileptics in a series of nationwide surveys between 1949 and 1979 (Caveness et al., 1974; Caveness and Gallup, 1980). The data indicate that over the past three decades there has been a reduction of prejudice toward people with epilepsy. These studies suggest, for instance, that fewer people today would object to their children playing with epileptics (from 43 percent in 1949 to 11 percent in 1979), and relatively fewer people think epilepsy is a form of insanity (from 41 percent to 8 percent). On the other hand, 20 percent of the population in 1979 did not agree with the statement epileptics "should be employed in jobs like other people." This 20 percent shortfall has remained virtually unchanged over the past two decades. More educated, better employed, younger, and urban people have displayed less prejudicial attitudes. A smaller study comparing public acceptance of epileptics to alcoholics and blind persons found that epileptics were more accepted than alcoholics but less so than the blind (Ries, 1977). This study asked people about their willingness to participate with epileptics in a variety of hypothetical situations. Acceptance was inversely related to social distance: 53 percent would not allow their child to marry a person with epilepsy; 26 percent did not want to rent a room to one; 11 percent would not want to work with one; 8 percent would not let an epileptic into their club, and 5 percent would not allow an epileptic in their neighborhood. Clearly, the most prejudice existed in the most intimate (marrying) and proximate (renting) situations. While other studies have shown more tolerance toward epileptics (e.g., Hauck, 1973; Caveness and Gallup, 1980), it is significant to find such a degree of prejudice toward any group of persons. The cost of prejudice is difficult to calculate, but it is safe to conclude that any impact it has on the quality of the lives of people with epilepsy would be negative.

Discrimination moves our attention to what people actually do, and in particular what they do toward individuals defined as members of some category or group. Discriminatory behavior may emerge informally, over time, or it may be produced by official policies, the intention of which may or may not be to effect such treatment. This discriminatory treatment, whatever its source and reasons for perpetuation, virtually always results in reduced opportunities for the target groups. In the case of epilepsy, employment is perhaps the most significant area of discrimination. In 1975, at least 23 percent of people with epilepsy were unemployed, compared to a national rate of 8.5 percent. This is a 14.5 percent excess in unemployment (Commission Report, 1978, Vol. II, Pt. 1).

Numerous studies (Wolfson, 1960; Schwartz, 1978; Hicks and Hicks, 1968, 1978) have demonstrated that employer discrimination is probably the largest factor in this excessive unemployment. Employers are often reluctant to hire people with epilepsy. Although attitudes seem to be improving (Schwartz, 1978, in Commission Report, 1978, Vol. II, Pt. I: 490), a seizure at work may still mean the immediate loss of a job. While employers may be hesitant to hire people with seizure disorders to operate hazardous machinery or drive vehicles, having epilepsy, if uncomplicated by other conditions, has little adverse effect on employee productivity or safety (Schwartz, 1978, in Commission Report). A Department of Labor study showed that persons with epilepsy had better safety records than other workers, and nearly all people with epilepsy are capable of some level of employment (*Federal Register* 42, no. 86 [May 4, 1977]: 22676). Until 1959, however, people with epilepsy were not hired for federal civil service positions and only recently have been allowed to serve in the armed forces.

Beyond unemployment, there is evidence that underemployment rates are even higher. For example, the 1975 national average weekly salary was $185; people with epilepsy earned $148.53 (Commission Report, 1978, Vol. I: 17). People with epilepsy are aware of this type of discrimination and attempt to control information to avoid it (see Chapter Seven). A nationwide survey estimated that one third of all people with epilepsy lie about their condition on job applications (National Epilepsy League, 1976). Since work is intimately linked with identity, for many, if not most people, such job discrimination amplifies identity problems and feelings of unworthiness.

Two other significant forms of discrimination involve obtaining insurance and a driver's license. Epilepsy is often considered a "high risk" category for insurance. People with epilepsy have only been able to obtain life insurance since World War II. A recent survey showed 52 percent of the respondents had difficulty securing life insurance; 40 percent had problems getting medical or hospital insurance; 37 percent, accident insurance; and 32 percent found it difficult to obtain automobile insurance (Commission Report, 1978, Vol. I: 104). The Epilepsy Foundation of America, in response to these problems, has begun offering specific life insurance policies.

Getting and keeping a driver's license can be among the most difficult problems for a person with epilepsy. Most states typically require a person to be seizure free (with or without medications) for one to two years before allowing them to receive a license. Physicians are asked to certify that a person has been seizure free (Epilepsy Foundation of America, 1976). This barrier is erected in the name of public safety, but epilepsy varies so greatly in terms of seizure warning time, occurrence of seizures (e.g., some people only have them in their sleep), and type and context of seizures, that casting such a wide net includes many people who could drive safely. Moreover, there is little if any systematic data to show the involvement of epileptic seizures in automobile accidents and fatalities. There is, in fact, some evidence to suggest this involvement is very low (Lennox and Lennox, 1960, Vol. 2: 972; Sullivan, 1981: 58). The irony here is that it is quite the opposite: about 20,000 Americans per year develop epilepsy *as a result* of injuries suffered in automobile accidents (Commission Report, 1978, Vol. I: 33). Restrictions on obtaining a driver's license become a very severe form of discrimination for people with epilepsy, not only because not driving makes people dependent on others, but because a driver's license is a major form of identification and a symbol of full-fledged adult competence.*

Over all, then, the social response to epilepsy has created a variety of barriers for those who have the disorder. Medical definitions and treatments have come to dominate the professional discourse about epilepsy. To a certain extent, public understanding of this medical reality has removed official barriers and reduced some of the more extreme public stereotypes and fears.

THE MEDICAL REALITY OF
EPILEPSY

Today the medical reality is the dominant social reality of epilepsy. Medicine and physicians have had primary ownership of epilepsy; prevalent stigma, prejudice, and discrimination to the contrary notwithstanding. In this section we review briefly the medical perspective, focusing on the issues of diagnosis, etiology, epidemiology, prognosis, and treatment. Since our major concern is with the social reality of epilepsy, we present the medical perspective as an important part of the social context with which people must contend.

DIAGNOSIS

Epilepsy is not considered a distinct disease, but rather a symptom. Physicians label most seizure disorders epilepsy, although researchers write about "the epilepsies."

---

*A few states, for example Washington and Ohio, recently eliminated the specific seizure-free time period requirement and substituted a statement from a physician that the individual is controlled adequately and thus able to drive safely (*National Spokesman*, June/July 1982: 8).

According to this view, seizures are produced by "intermittent electrochemical impulses in the brain" (HEW-NIH, 1975). A standard medical textbook defines epilepsy as follows: "A convulsive disorder is the expression of a sudden, excessive, disorderly discharge of neurons in either a structurally normal or diseased cortex. The discharge results in an almost instantaneous disturbance of sensation, loss of consciousness, convulsive movement, or some combination thereof" (Harrison, 1980: 131).

There are two related medical categorizations available for epilepsy, with some slight variation in terminology. The older and more well-known includes grand mal, petit mal, focal seizure patterns (psychomotor), and localized motor seizures (Jacksonian, focal motor, and contraversive). Many standard medical sources still use this typology and most people with epilepsy use these categories in describing their type of epilepsy. In recent years a newer classification has gained popularity, incorporating and superceding the older typology. Gastaut (1970) and Merlis (1970) have proposed classifications of "epileptic seizures" and the "epilepsies," respectively, that have received widespread attention and official endorsement (see Commission Report 1978, Vol. I: 20–21). They include the following major categories: "Generalized Seizures or Epilepsies," "Partial Seizures or Epilepsies," and "Unclassifiable."

These are complex categories subsuming a variety of movements and internal processes. The "partial" epilepsies include all those typical conditions in which only a segment of the brain—and corresponding overt movements— is involved. Incorporated here are the long-used seizure types of "psychomotor," "Jacksonian," "focal," "local," and "temporal lobe." Typical movements in the partial epilepsies are localized muscle contractions, problems in speaking, tactile sensations in various parts of the body, distorted sight and impaired consciousness, auditory hallucinations, and sometimes repetitive movements of the mouth, arms, hands, and legs. Generalized epilepsy, by contrast, appears to affect the entire body. Its two major sub-types are grand mal and petit mal—translated as "little" and "great" sickness.

Reflecting the growing medical dissatisfaction with classic petit and grand mal labels (they are increasingly considered "misleading" and stigmatizing), the new classi-fications place these terms in parentheses after the pre-ferred "absences" and "tonic-clonic." Absence, or petit mal, seizures are typified by the physical, intellectual, and affective appearance of someone who is "away" or "ab-sent" from the social environment. Such behaviors are gen-erally brief in duration, lasting from a few seconds to per-haps a minute, and involve a stare, preoccupied glance, rhythmic blinking, muscle jerking, some "automatic" move-ments, such as lip-smacking, chewing and picking at clothes or body. Considerably more dramatic and visible is the tonic-clonic or grand mal seizure. The person so classified loses consciousness and falls to the floor in sometimes vio-lent convulsive movements. This may include involuntary salivation, gnashing of teeth, and incontinence. These sei-zures last somewhat longer than either petit mal or local-ized episodes and are often followed by a period of deep sleep. About half the people who have grand mal seizures experience a warning or "aura."

Grand mal or tonic-clonic seizures alone are the single most common type (roughly 50 percent of those diag-nosed), followed by combinations of grand mal with psy-chomotor or petit mal (25 percent), and other forms of minor epilepsy only (including psychomotor, 20 percent) (Commission Report, 1978, Vol. I: 21–22). In from 3 to 8 percent of adults with epilepsy, an event known as "status epilepticus" occurs (Commission Report, 1978, Vol. II, Pt. I: 163). This is a situation in which the person has one seizure after another in quick succession. It is considered to be a medical emergency and can lead to disability and death.

ETIOLOGY

The causes of epilepsy are often unclear. When no causal factor can be identified, the condition is labeled idiopathic epilepsy. As we discussed earlier, in a small number of cases there seems to be hereditary predisposition to the disorder. When epilepsy is identified as symptomatic or acquired, this means it is possible to attribute cause. The major known causes of epilepsy are perinatal factors, infection (especially in early childhood), and trauma (head injury, especially from automobile accidents). There is some evidence that laws mandating seat belts, safety helmets for motorcyclists, and enforcement of the 55 mph speed limit have measurably reduced the incidence of epilepsy (Commission Report, 1978, Vol. IV: 170–175). One study only could identify epilepsy's cause in 23.6 percent of the cases, leaving the majority with unknown origins (Hauser and Kurland, 1975).

EPIDEMIOLOGY

Epidemiology is the study of the distribution of disease in a population. It is an important method for locating potential causal factors and the extent of the disease. Because epilepsy is stigmatized and often kept secret, it is difficult to collect accurate epidemiological data. The Epilepsy Commission Report used the following figures as minimums. The estimated incidence of epilepsy in the United States is 46.7 per 100,000, or roughly 100,000 new cases each year. Hauser and Kurland (1975), in a study of Rochester, Minnesota, from 1935 to 1967, using very conservative criteria to define a seizure disorder, found 3.9 cases per 1,000 population at one year of age and 9.1 cases per 1,000 population at age seventy. Using 1970 population age-adjusted prevalence data, they concluded that 6.25 of every 1,000 people had epilepsy. The Epilepsy Commission estimated that one percent of the population, about two million Americans, had epilepsy (Commission Report 1978, Vol. I: 17). They estimated that 20–25 percent of these people are unidentified epileptics and have had no medical contact (Vol. IV: 88–89). There is some evidence from another study of Rochester, Minnesota, that the incidence of epilepsy in children under age twenty is declining, probably due to the general improvement in care given to mothers and children (see Commission Report, Vol. II, Pt. 1: 242). Epilepsy can occur at any age but is most common in the first twenty years.

PROGNOSIS AND TREATMENT

With a few exceptions, adults who get epilepsy have it for the rest of their lives. Childhood epilepsy, however, displays various remission patterns. One recent study showed that about 40 percent of children studied experienced remission for four years (Sofijanov, 1982); another, showing an even higher remission rate, concluded that children who do not have additional risk factors, "have an excellent chance of remaining seizure-free after the withdrawal of convulsant drugs" (Thurston et al., 1982). In general, however, there is a poor prognosis for long-range freedom from seizures other than with childhood epilepsy (Commission Report, 1978, Vol. II, Pt. 9).

Although "cure" is rare, "control" is common. The prognosis in terms of control with anticonvulsant medication is quite good. The Commission Report (1978, Vol. II, Pt. 1: 491) concludes: "About half of the epileptic population will achieve complete seizure control, and an additional 35 percent can achieve good seizure control (three or four seizures a year)." This means that 85 percent of people with epilepsy can reduce significantly the number of seizures experienced by using these medications. Lennox and Lennox (1960: 34) reflect these estimates when they claim, "The emancipation of the epileptic by the physician began some three hundred years ago and has proceeded with progressively increasing success." But this "emancipation" is far from complete. Epilepsy remains a morally tainted disorder and society's response still resonates with prejudice and discrimination. And, as we have noted, physicians have reinforced as well as reduced the stigma of epilepsy.

Even in the face of the dominant medical reality and associated improvements in seizure control, epilepsy, like leprosy and veneral disease, continues to be a stigmatized illness. In spite of epilepsy's nearly total medicalization, the disorder remains connected with social condemnation and stigma and subject to discrimination. This seems to be the case in non-Western societies as well (e.g., Danesi et al., 1981), although rare exceptions exist where epileptics have been seen as blessed by the spirits (see Watson, 1981). In American society overt discrimination appears to be decreasing, but the stigma potential of epilepsy remains. One promising finding is that 63 percent of Americans said they know someone who has epilepsy, and 59 percent reported to have seen a seizure (Caveness and Gallup, 1980). This suggests a decrease in stigma-induced secrecy among people with epilepsy and an increased potential for a discourse between epileptics and various others. This may lead ultimately to an elimination of the social barriers and the historical moral residues with which people have had and continue to live.

THREE
Discovery

In one sense, the story of what it is like to have epilepsy, or cancer, or diabetes, or any other illness begins with medical diagnosis. People come under scrutiny of a physician and are told that they "have" this or that disease or disorder. But medical diagnosis is not usually the origin of illness experience and sometimes does not come at the beginning of people's involvement with doctors. Our own experiences with illness tell us that often long before going to the doctor, we "know something is wrong." We ache, "feel bad," are unable to do things we usually do, or experience a jarring sign that some aspect of our bodies or minds is not "as it should be."* To understand the experience of epilepsy, we

---

* This prediagnosis period is the object of the illness behavior research discussed in Chapter One.

must consider what happens before people take their problems to professionals. Accordingly, we begin our account at our respondents' first remembered "signs of trouble."

DEFINITIONS, DIAGNOSIS, AND DISCOVERY

When we asked our respondents how they first found out they had epilepsy, almost all said, "I had a seizure." Some went on to tell how this first seizure, usually dramatic and sometimes causing physical injury, led quickly to the hospital or doctor's office, an array of "tests," and a diagnosis of epilepsy within a matter of hours or days. One man recalled such experience at age seventeen:

> I was in debate [in high school] and I was judging a debate between two sophomores. I stood up to give criticisms and decisions and I had a seizure, and got taken to the hospital. Didn't know what the hell was goin' on. Thought I was gonna die or something. Really hadn't had anything to indicate I had a problem of that sort. Stayed in the hospital for a couple of days, while I think they did all the normal things to discover if I had brain tumors or . . . brain damage, or . . . I was insane [laughs]. They just determined I had that amorphous thing called epilepsy and started to give me drugs regularly.

A young woman described her "first seizure" that led to diagnosis at age nineteen:

> I was just sitting there and I was reading a magazine . . . and I had had a headache earlier, and all of a sudden I just started feeling really funny. I was chewing gum and something told me that I had to get that gum out of my mouth. My sister-in-law was sitting across the room and I was trying to say something to her and then I was out. The next thing I knew I woke up and I was in the hospital and I was scared. I didn't know what was wrong, and they were telling me, you know, well it could be a brain tumor or it could be an

aneurysm and all this and they did all these weird
tests and finally they did an EEG and they said it was
epilepsy.

In each of these and similar stories, what people only later
came to recognize as a "seizure" was defined by those
around them as a medical emergency, they were taken immediately to the hospital or to a doctor, and soon thereafter
medically diagnosed. This kind of experience, in which first
seizure and diagnosis are close together in time, was not
typical. In fact, of the eighty people we interviewed, only
28, or 35 percent, recalled such a quick connection between a first, unanticipated seizure, and medical diagnosis.

Most people's stories remind us that diagnosis is more
than simply medical labeling or categorization. In its most
general sense, diagnosis is a process of definition that includes not just "official" medical labels, but laboratory and
clinical evidence, highly-trained professional specialists
and more (see Blaxter, 1976, 1978). An insight from some
sociologists of deviance (e.g., Becker, 1963; Kitsuse, 1962)
can expand our understanding of diagnosis beyond medical labeling and help us to think of it more as a definitional
process involving a variety of participants: the ill person,
family members, friends, work associates, various professional or service workers, in addition to physicians and
other (usually neglected) medical personnel (cf. Freidson,
1970). This expanded view allows us to consider seriously
our respondents' stories as windows on the experience of
diagnosis rather than discounting them as "idiosyncratic,"
or irrelevant "overreactions" ascribed to ignorance (cf.
Locker, 1981).

MAKING THE STRANGE
FAMILIAR:
LAY DEFINITIONS

What our respondents, after diagnosis, came to call seizures are made up of a great variety of feelings, sensations,
movements, sounds, and sights (see Chapter Five). In fact,

these "things," as some people called them, do not become "seizures," until someone, usually a physician or medical specialist, actually uses this word to describe them. "Strange feelings," "headaches," "spaciness," "blackouts," and "dizzy spells" then *become* "seizures," seen retrospectively as evidence that "something was wrong all along." Past experience is reinterpreted in light of the present diagnosis. Having a name for these frightening and always inexplicable experiences can be comforting.

When a first seizure did not lead quickly to diagnosis, the most common response was to try to make sense of what was happening. Much social science research shows that one common way people bring order to these "disordered" situations is to bring familiar frames of reference or meaning to the problematic event. Some of our respondents saw their feelings and movements, including loss of consciousness, falling to the ground, and muscular convulsions, as, if not exactly normal, at least something that could be explained by specific features of the situation.

Research and writing on deviance again can help us understand how our respondents and others made these prediagnosis events and feelings familiar. Sociologists have used the terms "normalization" and "neutralization" to refer to how people make sense of conduct and situations seen as out of the ordinary or as violating expectations (Yarrow et al., 1955; Sykes and Matza, 1957). They found that people accommodated their own and others' unusual behavior by developing conventional and/or alternate definitions of such conduct (see also Waddell, 1982). This observation can be extended to include how people make sense of and explain bodily aches, pains, unusual feelings, and events. For instance, when we "feel warm" or flushed we hypothesize that "something is wrong," take our temperature, find it is 102 degrees F., conclude we were correct in our hypothesis, perhaps develop some "reason" for it, and take steps to reduce our temperature. To *normalize* such events would be to say, in effect, "nothing is *really* wrong"; that such a temperature is within the realm of what might be expected; it is "normal," in short, not problematic (due, for instance, to recent "stressful" situations). Our respondents described a range of such normalizing definitions for the first physical signs of epilepsy, seizures, or impending seizures.*

We asked one 28-year-old woman, who had just been medically diagnosed, if she had any previous seizures. She said:

> Not that I knew. I didn't know what they were. You know, I talked . . . I knew people that had epilepsy and, uh . . . I just, it wasn't like the seizures that they had had. I've had headaches ever since I was little-bitty, and I just, it's somethin' that I was gonna live with. It got to the point where these "things," I didn't call them seizures at that time, got to the point where I was havin' like ten to twelve a day. And everybody said, you know, "You better go and . . ." I would get real short of breath, like I was gonna pass out . . . get real shaky and just sick to my stomach. But I never passed out.

One man diagnosed at eighteen said that after he knew what his seizures were, he could recall having them while growing up. It was "like daydreaming," and his parents treated them as intentional:

> Besides . . . before that [diagnosis], I'd always had the tendency to roll my eyes back in my head . . . to kind of fade out for a while. But I thought that was nothing, but they . . . I guess they call them petit mal? I'd lose consciousness for a while. I wasn't really conscious of it and any time anybody would notice it was when the family was all together at the dinner table and I,

---

*Whether what is called the "aura" should be considered as part of the seizure or a separate event is an issue in medical discussion. For our purposes, we treat all "strange feelings," including the actual seizure, as part of what we call "prediagnosis seizures," since they all constitute "problems" to be explained by the person experiencing them.

> I'd be like daydreaming for a while and then I'd roll
> my eyes back and they'd go, "Stop that!" and I'd go,
> "Stop what?," y'know, I didn't know what I was doin'.

Family members had complained about this behavior "for quite a while, probably as far back as junior high." When asked what his parents and others thought he was doing, he said, "I don't know. They just thought it was strange, they just [said], 'Stop that!'" He never thought to ask about going to a doctor.

Sometimes such normalizing was accomplished by relating the experience to routine bodily changes or processes. One woman said she began having "these strange feelings" following a head injury while ice skating. They got progressively stronger until finally she had a grand mal seizure and was diagnosed. In describing her feelings, she said: "Well, I had no way to explain what they were. I called them dizzy spells, but actually they just, I don't know what they were, uh, it's called the aura, you know, and it would just spread all over me." How did she make sense of these feelings, and did she have concerns about them?:

> Well, yes, but my parents didn't, so I thought, well,
> maybe it's just me, y'know, and I just put it off. I didn't
> think too much about it, and it seemed like they came
> along with the menstrual cycle, and I just put it off
> with that. My parents put it off with that. By sum-
> mertime I was having them every day . . . until finally
> in the fall this aura just went into a grand mal.

In these and similar cases, unusual feelings and movements were defined explicitly, as in "daydreaming," or implicitly, in conjunction with menstruation or stress, as typical components of the person's conduct or situation.

When people create *neutralizing* definitions they accommodate such experience by, in effect, "working around it": by discounting it as unworthy of attention, although perhaps inconvenient. Our respondents neutralized their strange feelings and experiences by concluding they were insignificant. One man said, "I just decided it was nothing." Another said he had "probably a dozen blackouts" before he went to the doctor. A woman had several minor auto accidents because of "blackouts" before going to the doctor. These cases also illustrate the importance of others as collaborators in such definitional work. "Everybody" urged the woman to go see a doctor; the young man's family treated his "daydreaming" and eye rolling as willful inattention and orneriness; the woman's parents defined her seizures as part of their daughter's "natural" menstruation, and so on.

For those diagnosed as children, parents were the most important collaborators, often assuming full control of their child's understanding of what was happening. When they noticed something "unusual," and particularly if it was obvious or repeated, parents usually sought professional medical opinion. Some respondents, however, told stories about parents who delayed taking them to a doctor, even though these parents had witnessed recurrent bizarre conduct. We address such diverse parental involvement in detail in the next chapter.

MEDICAL UNCERTAINTY: DELAYING DISCOVERY

Parents were not the only collaborators who delayed the discovery of epilepsy. Physicians themselves, even when consulted specifically for the strange feelings and behaviors described, sometimes offered normalizing and neutralizing definitions, such as "normal under the circumstances," or "probably a one-time occurrence" and "nothing to worry about." Even when people sought and received medical attention for these problems, they were not necessarily given a diagnosis of epilepsy (cf. Stewart and Sullivan, 1982). Becoming a patient does not always lead to discovering "what is wrong." There is some evidence, moreover, that doctors themselves may harbor many of the same stereotypes and misconceptions of people with epilepsy that are found in the general population (Beran et al., 1981; Beran and Read, 1983).

Nearly all people who have had seizures are eventually sent to a hospital for tests, which may include EEGs, x-rays, brain scans and other components of a neurological workup. While it is possible to take these tests as an outpatient, many respondents said they spent anywhere from a night to a week in the hospital while doctors determined the diagnosis and appropriate treatment (much of this time may be given to monitoring the patient's reaction to medications).

In other cases, diagnosis is not so straightforward and there is considerable uncertainty. Contrary to popular thinking, such uncertainty is a typical part of medical practice, perhaps most clear in diagnosis itself (e.g., Conrad, 1976: 51–69). As sociologist David Mechanic (1968: 23) notes: "Medical knowledge is a mixture of scientifically precise facts and clinical impressions, leaving much room for medical uncertainty and individual variation to manifest itself in regard to problems patients present to doctors." A seizure disorder like epilepsy is not a clear-cut disease with uniform signs and symptoms. The diagnosis is the product of clinical medical judgment based on the results of various "tests" and the patient's reported symptoms. At times, doctors have difficulty making a diagnosis or finding a satisfactory treatment, so they try different hypotheses and solutions, including normalizing and neutralizing definitions (see Hopkins and Scambler, 1977).

A young college student told of going to his doctor for "fainting spells." His doctor said he was "just homesick" and suggested he could control it if he tried. One 33-year-old man remembered momentary blackouts while in junior high school, about which he did nothing. He had his first seizure while on a senior trip and was "run through every kind of test" the doctor "could think of, and he could not find a thing wrong with me." He went on to college, where he promptly had a seizure, "chipped a tooth and banged myself up a little bit," and was soon thereafter diagnosed at a university medical center. A woman said she began "passing out" at age fourteen. She had been diagnosed as having several other medical conditions, including anemia, low blood pressure, heart problems, and cerebral palsy. Her doctors attributed her fainting to one of these other conditions and did not pursue it as a sign of epilepsy. One young man told a story that represents the experience of many respondents. He described his first seizure:

> Well, it was weird because I went to school and everything was, y'know, normal, but then I went to homeroom and at the time I didn't know but now I look back on it, I was totally unconscious to everything. People would say, "Bob," and I wouldn't even answer. I went to first hour, which was choir, ninth grade choir, and I couldn't remember any of the words to the songs. I couldn't do anything and I couldn't remember my locker combination, you name it. I just was really goofy. . . . Then we went to second hour and I remember I was lookin' at this kid's ninth grade pictures, and the next thing I remember was waking up in an ambulance. . . . I stayed in the hospital I guess a couple of days. I remember I slept for about a day and a half right afterwards and they sent me home and they said it was stress.

We asked him if while in the hospital anyone told him he might have epilepsy. He said no, but that he remembered his school nurse saying to someone at the time that he had had a convulsion. He recalled no tests being done during his visit to the hospital; "they just said, 'You're rested up now. Go home. It was probably stress.'" We asked when he remembered hearing the word "epilepsy" used to describe his experiences:

> Well, after the first one the word epilepsy never came up. I never even heard it, you know, as far as nobody ever said it could be or sounds like epilepsy. My parents never said anything, so I just went on, you know,

normal, and three weeks later, bam, the same thing. It
was within half an hour of the first one. I remember I
couldn't remember my locker combination then,
either.

Not having the diagnostic label to apply, he and his parents
were perplexed by this second episode. He said: "You just
don't think about it [that you might have something]. I
mean it just doesn't go through your mind that you're that
way. You just slough it off and you say, [about not remem-
bering things], 'Ah, darn it.'" After this second seizure his
parents called their family doctor, who referred them first
to one neurologist and then another at a major medical
center. There, after more tests, he was told he was "very
prone to convulsions," that they could be controlled by
medication, and that he was to start taking Dilantin. He
noted in passing, "come to think of it, they never actually
used the word 'epilepsy.'"

A 27-year-old woman told of a childhood of "passing
out" that was always attributed to her being "overly heated"
and "excited." Finally, at age twenty-four she was examined
by a doctor who told her she had epilepsy. She said, "They
figured out that I was an epileptic from birth." She told us
she had seen "literally twenty-seven doctors" before being
diagnosed: "Everytime I would pass out they would make
me go get another physical and they just kept sayin', 'Oh,
she was just over-heated.'"

Some of our older respondents told stories of prediagnosis medical definitions that seemed closer to folk than to
scientific medicine. A 52-year-old woman said she had had
several seizures before being diagnosed twenty years earlier. Doctors said her first seizure was the product of a
"toxic pregnancy." The second her physician ascribed to
"hot weather" and that it was a typical "housewife's complaint." Another woman, fifty-four, began having seizures in
her early twenties: "Something would come over me and I
felt like I was going to die. And so I doctored and the doctor told me, he says, 'Drink some coffee.' And I says, 'Well, I

never drink coffee.' And he said, 'Drink coffee. That might help you enough.'" She said that the feelings "got worse" and "it just got to where I would bite my tongue and I would black clear out."

Sometimes patients received diagnoses other than epilepsy. The most common alternate diagnosis was some vague kind of "emotional," "psychological," or "psychiatric" problem to explain the strange feelings and conduct. Our data suggest, but do not make clear, that such diagnoses followed various kinds of "difficulty" with parents or others, such that the unusual behavior was seen as "bad" or disruptive, and willful. All of these stories of alternate psychiatric or "emotional" diagnoses, moreover, came from women. This is perhaps not surprising in that research shows women to be more "at risk" for such affective disorder diagnoses than men (Dohrenwend and Dohrenwend, 1974, 1976). Marcia Millman (1976), while studying medical practice in a large teaching hospital, found that when patient complaints persisted in the absence of a firm diagnosis of a physiological disorder, some physicians concluded the patient suffered from a psychiatric problem. One woman recalled such an experience:

> I had problems talking, especially at the dinner table. If my parents asked me a direct question I would get nervous and wouldn't answer them and they would get upset. Also, in school I would get nervous and wouldn't answer and they would get upset. I wasn't actually having seizures at the time but I was having blackouts.

She said finally she was taken to a neurologist, had tests and was diagnosed. Prior to that her family doctor had suggested to her parents that "it might be a psychiatric type thing." She added: "I really didn't know what to think."

A 21-year-old woman said she had "fainting spells" since she was a freshman in college but was not diagnosed as having epilepsy until three years later. During this time her doctors insisted her problem was "psychosomatic."

And another woman received therapy at a mental health unit for a year after a series of "blackouts":

> I really didn't think of me having epilepsy for a long time. It was never talked about as epilepsy. They [her general practitioner] first thought I had a psychological problem because of the death of my husband and I was blacking out. They sent me to a psychiatrist, a psychologist, for over a year. It was never regarded as epilepsy . . . it was just an emotional thing. It wasn't until [later] when I went to [a major medical center] that they used the word "epilepsy."

In each of these cases respondents presented to doctors complaints that were normalized as understandable under the circumstances; neutralized, as something unknown yet nevertheless of little lasting significance, or taken as grounds for various diagnoses other than epilepsy, most commonly some vague kind of "psychological problem." While it certainly is possible that these physician-offered definitions were appropriate, the point is that even when these people did go to a physician, it in some cases took quite some time before they finally discovered epilepsy.

SELF DIAGNOSIS AND PESSIMISTIC ACCOUNTS

Given the time separating the initial perceptions of "trouble" and the ultimate diagnosis for some of our respondents, coupled with a sustained sense of "not knowing what is happening," it is not surprising to find a small number of people who said they actually diagnosed themselves. Sometimes this was done by systematic reading and study, stimulated by what they heard physicians or nurses say about them and their situation. One 49-year-old woman had seizures since she was about fifteen but discovered her epilepsy only at age thirty-five, after reading an article in *Reader's Digest* magazine. She had seen many physicians, taken Dilantin for years, but had never been told, either by her parents or a doctor, that she had epilepsy. In fact, no name was given her condition by a physician until about five years after she discovered it herself, when she said a neurologist wrote "classical epilepsy" on a consultation report to her family doctor.

Sometimes such self-diagnoses were made on the basis of experience with family members who also had epilepsy, or on the basis of specific remarks from others. After suffering a serious fall and head injury at about age twelve, one woman said: "I would start waking up and my tongue would be sore. I knew that symptom because my brother has epilepsy. So, that's when I started suspecting it." Entertaining such a definition about one's self was sometimes done grudgingly. One woman told of how, as a college student, she

> met a girl that was an epileptic and she really thought
> I was one, just by the way I couldn't stand the lights.
> And she kept tellin' me I was one and I kept callin'
> her a liar, cuz that was the *last* thing I wanted to be.
> And when she kept sayin' I was, you know, it really
> started to bug me, so I kinda broke off being friends
> with her. I'd seen her have a seizure . . . and I defi-
> nitely didn't wanna be one! I just kept tellin' her my
> problems were not the same as hers.

We asked another woman, who had been diagnosed just recently, if anyone had ever suggested to her before that time that she might have epilepsy. She said:

> Yeah, the swimming instructor last year at camp, gave
> me this book on epilepsy. And, all the symptoms that
> were there, I seemed to have. And she kept sayin',
> "Well, why don't you get this checked out?' I'd say,
> 'Well, uh, no. That's okay." But in the back of my mind,
> something was, you know, I thought maybe it was but
> I didn't wanna bring it up. She had seen me pass out a
> couple of times . . . and she thought I was real spacy.

In such situations, we see the conjunction of suggested diagnoses by others and suspicions held by the individual that serve to produce both more thinking and, in some cases, "research." For instance, one man diagnosed at twelve said his physicians intentionally avoided the terms "epilepsy" and "seizures." His neurologist called his seizures "spells." When in college he went to another doctor for a physical examination. A nurse asked him about any medication he was taking; he said he told her and "immediately the nurse says to me, 'Are you epileptic?' And I said, 'No, but I had had a brain tumor,' because that's the way, you know, I'd kinda learned to explain it." This nurse was the first person to use the word epilepsy to refer to his condition. He said the encounter "made me more curious." Subsequently, he asked pharmacy-student friends about his medication and the conditions for which it was prescribed. He then "concluded this is a form of epilepsy. And so I talked to my parents and said, 'Why didn't anyone ever say this?'"

Beyond normalizing, neutralizing, and denying, another way in which we can "make sense" of problematic situations is to construe them as indicating impending disaster—in short, to imagine "the worst." We can "pessimize." In the face of both their own uncertainty and their physicians', coupled with knowledge of things doctors actually mentioned, such as "brain tumor" and "blood clot," some respondents pursued these possibilities as logical and likely explanations. One man's comments provide a sense of how ambiguity, medical uncertainty, and a sense of gravity about one's condition can easily produce results that make coping difficult:

Nobody would tell you things and you'd look up things on your own. You'd hear doctors talking about things, you'd pick out certain words and, you know, you're a little paranoid if you have something and you don't know what it is. And I'd been hearing things and so like I didn't know what a brain tumor was. It didn't mean anything to me, so I went and looked it up on my own and I got a lot of misinformation on my own. I got a lot of strange ideas on my own. I figured the reason they wouldn't tell me was because I was going to die and they didn't have the nerve to tell me that. And, you know, that sounds strange to me even, but at that time it was serious.

That patients come to such conclusions about their condition and prognosis should be seen more as a product of context than of personality or "suggestibility." We do, after all, place great stock in medical expertise and its capacity to render quick, clear diagnoses, and implement wonderful, increasingly technologically sophisticated solutions. Such expectations seem to set the stage for seeing medical ambiguity and delay as particularly ominous, portending grave news that is being "held back" for its jarring impact. Some who found themselves in such situations reasoned that "after all these tests, if they don't know or aren't telling, it must be very bad."

Such pessimizing can even come before an extended period of seemingly fruitless doctor and hospital visits. As we noted earlier, when people perceive body and mind problems they seek answers. This does not always mean immediately contacting a doctor or medical professional. We have little data on lay theorizing beyond such nonmedical accounts as those discussed here (see Chapter Five for a discussion of lay theories of seizure incidence and frequency). One might suspect that such "research" prior to contacting a doctor is more common among people who have access to medical handbooks of both the popular and professional varieties than among those who do not. Those who have learned to handle uncertainty by reading and otherwise seeking out relevant information from family members and friends might also be in this category. It is likely, then, that attempts at developing lay explanations prior to or even in conjunction with contacting medical professionals might vary by social class (see Koos, 1954). As the above quote suggests, however, obtaining such information does not necessarily produce either more peace of mind or effective treatment.

For the most part, pessimizing seemed to be associated with a rather lengthy period of medical consultation, preceded by or coincidental with ongoing "uncontrolled" seizures. Many reported this to be profoundly frustrating. One woman said she had concluded the worst and, after a protracted time with no firm answers, was about to take drastic steps to bring closure to her history:

> I had built up in my mind by the time I went to the doctor [a neurologist, the last physician of several she had consulted] that I probably had a brain tumor or I was . . . there for a while I thought maybe I was . . . going crazy, you know, just to myself. Like I said, it had been going on for five years, and I just was to the point if I hadn't gone to [that] doctor when I did, I'da probably done something that I would have regretted. I was just so terribly frustrated by all of this goin' on . . . and mostly [with] doctors that I have had confidence in sayin', "Oh, I don't know what it is," and, y'know, nobody suggestin' that maybe I go see a neurologist.

While this woman and some others did come to such pessimistic judgments about their problems and futures "on their own," it is important to point out that this was accomplished by drawing on what others, including physicians, had said and done. We do not suggest that these people's doctors were necessarily wrong or made mistakes, but that in situations such as these, where fear, ambiguity, great expectations of experts, and dire possibilities come together, pessimistic conclusions and courses of action based on them are one way that people attempt to cope.

SOC/ ANOTHRO

THE IMPACT OF A MEDICAL
LABEL

To discover that one has epilepsy is to face a social reality over which one will have, at most, only partial control. Anxiety and ambiguity aside, when "blackouts," "headaches," and "spaciness" become "seizures," and when the
cause is something called "epilepsy" or a "seizure disorder" certified by a medical expert, one moves to a set of
meanings, prescribed courses of conduct, and interaction
that alters experience, past, present, and future. Whether
or not people actually used the term "epileptic" to describe themselves (many said they did not), to have a medical diagnosis applied is to think and to have others think of
us in a new way, as an instance of a type—a "case."

Michael Balint (1972) suggests that upon diagnosis, patients move out of the "unorganized" stage of illness into
one involving order and a prescribed course of action. It
should be clear, however, that it is not so much a move
from disorder to order, but rather from a set of meanings
typical of lay and commonsense experience to one pre-
sided over by medical experts and a medical culture. When
we take our complaints and problems to experts we give
up a degree of control. By putting ourselves in professional
hands we agree, often quite tacitly, to accept the legitimacy of the review and judgment provided. Moreover,
since the medical establishment and its culture have such
popular and official warrant, these professional definitions
of us operate not only within hospital and clinic walls but
throughout the society. When people discovered they had
epilepsy, most began to think about themselves and the social realities discussed in Chapter Two.

We specifically asked our respondents what they
thought and how they felt when they discovered this new
"fact" about themselves. Most said they "really didn't know
what it was"; they had had little if any prior experience

with epilepsy. Some said they never even had heard the word. When people knew little or nothing of epilepsy, discovery seemed to be less traumatic. This was not simply a function of age. While those diagnosed as young children often recalled it as "not so terrible," adults who received their diagnoses against a background of ignorance expressed the same sentiments. One man who had discovered his epilepsy at age seven said: "I didn't know what it was. It didn't really shake me up too bad. At that age, kids don't, you know, get shook up by too much anyhow." Another said, "I don't think I really realized the potential nature of it" at age seventeen. He explained his "mild reaction" to discovery by calling himself "naïve" about "people's perceptions":

> I guess one of the things that may have relieved me of
> some of the pressures is that I didn't really associate
> epilepsy with . . . with anything particularly negative
> in terms of people's perceptions. I was pretty naïve
> about what it was, y'know, about how some people
> might perceive it. I didn't realize, for example, the ex-
> tent to which people are frightened by a seizure. . . . I
> didn't really realize those things. I didn't understand
> what people's perceptions, I should say some people's
> perceptions, were.

Our respondents soon learned many of the historical and social realities of epilepsy. A woman said when she found out at nineteen she had epilepsy, "I didn't know much about it . . . and then I started learning more and I found out how everyone else thought it was so awful."

Knowing little of epilepsy, but with a growing sense it was "something serious," respondents sometimes heightened rather than reduced these fears with their research efforts. A man diagnosed at sixteen said:

> I guess I didn't know anything about epilepsy. I was
> sixteen and never even heard of it. And it was kind of
> a shock because I decided I would find out what it
> was and the first thing I read about was when they

used to burn people that had epilepsy. I thought, "Wait a minute. I ain't gonna tell anybody about this." I guess from the very beginning I had a lot of misconceptions about what it was, a lot of misinformation, because the doctors weren't volunteering any . . . probably because they figured I wouldn't understand it anyway.

The theme of inadequate information about epilepsy, particularly at the time of discovery, ran through most of our interviews (see Chapter Eight for a more detailed discussion of problems associated with information). Yet while our respondents said they knew few facts about it as a medical condition, they soon came to see epilepsy as a new moral weight they had to carry. A very few said they had heard public service announcements or other public education efforts. One man said he knew what epilepsy was because he had lived in a state that had a "very active chapter" of the Epilepsy Foundation of America. Another said "[I know] there are medications I could be on to keep me from doing anything." Interestingly enough, however, he specifically mentioned seeing a "commercial" about epilepsy (presumably one of the announcements distributed by the EFA) and added "I thought about a commercial I had seen . . . that sometimes employment is hard to get if you have epilepsy." The announcement, aside from its intent, told him epilepsy might be a bar to getting or keeping a job, even though it should not be. He said, "I thought, 'What am I gonna do when I get a job? Think I'll lie.'" A woman said that at the time of her diagnosis she had heard of epilepsy once. "I think I was in fourth grade and we were told there was a boy in class that had epilepsy and that if he ever had a seizure we were supposed to run out of the room. Well, I had terrible fantasies of what happened to this poor kid and it really singled him out."

Such stories testify to how messages and actions, even those intended to have the opposite impact, can convey an image of epilepsy as something stigmatizing, undesirable, even terrible. To the extent that our respondents had learned of such meanings, their blissful ignorance gave way to apprehension about how others would see them and treat them.

Some respondents said they were "shocked" to learn of their condition, usually meaning that they had had some idea, usually negative, about epilepsy or people with this condition. One man said, "I was kinda shocked. I've always thought, you know, those people were different, but when I . . . it was kind of contradictory." A woman said when her doctor told her, "I was kind of numb, in a way. It didn't really hit me until after I had gotten out of the hospital. What they said was just like so shocking to me that everything else just didn't register." One of the most extreme negative reactions came from a woman whose parents had concealed the diagnosis from her for several months, during which time she continued to have seizures. She said when she found out,

I tried to commit suicide. I tried to take an overdose of the drugs I was on. I felt like some unclean spirit had walked in the door. I mean, I felt . . . uh, an oddball. Because nobody would communicate to me what it was about . . . I felt a great stigma attached to it.

Beyond vague negative feelings and apprehensions about what epilepsy might mean in their lives, a number of people said their major concern was "all the things I couldn't do" because of it. These "don'ts" were sometimes conveyed by the diagnosing physician or, more commonly, by parents wanting to be sure to protect their children and to keep them from harm's way. One man said: "First thing was they told me everything I can't do. I'm not supposed to get tired. I'm not supposed to drink. I'm not supposed to get over-exerted. And I said to myself, 'Man, there goes my life down the drain.'" Another young man, diagnosed at fourteen, said:

I began to think about the things I couldn't do. I knew from that day forward my parents were always going to be a lot more, you know, "Well, I'm gonna camp out tonight," you know, "Well are you sure you better?" You know, that sort of thing. I never thought of anything except about the pleasures that it would bum up. The doctors told me to look at the bright side of it. You at least can't be drafted.

Driving restrictions were among the concerns most often mentioned by adolescent respondents, particularly the males. One young man said that when the doctor told him at age fourteen about having epilepsy, "I thought, 'This is all I need, they're going to take my license away now,' 'cuz I heard them talk about that." He went on:

They told me you have to go a year without a seizure [before you can drive]. I started to cry then, to myself. I was in a room by myself and I just couldn't take it. . . . It was hard to accept. The hardest part was the driving, not being able to drive and get around, to have to have someone haul you around all the time.

The young man who discovered his epilepsy at fourteen, said:

I do remember the first time I realized that there was something wrong that could affect me was when the doctor or one of his residents asked me how old I was. I told him and he said, "Well, that means you're going to be up to drive real soon." I said, yes. He said, "Well, you know the state has a law that you have to be seizure-free for a year," and I thought, "Well, now, *wait*. What are you saying?" I mean, you know, "Hold it!" and at the time I kind of thought that there may be something more to this than I had thought.

These and similar comments make it clear that the most difficult part of discovering epilepsy was confronting its social meanings. Those who had little or no idea of these meanings described reactions that were mild. Those who said they knew epilepsy was a medical condition for which one could take controlling medication reacted to epilepsy as a "normal medical problem." To the extent, however, that people knew or soon came to know of the stigma and social restrictions that surround epilepsy, discovery brought a whole new set of problems. They were now, suddenly, "officially" people with epilepsy, "epileptics;" it had become a reality of their lives and selves with which they would have to contend.

Another common reaction was a sense of "relief" to learn it was epilepsy rather than something worse. This relief comes in the context of the optimism inherent in medical definition and diagnosis, namely, that "something can be done about it." Even those who experienced discovery as a shocking revelation said at last they "knew what it was" and that this knowing brought an end to troubling questions and speculation.

So discovery had its brighter side, one that highlights precisely the shift Balint's (1972) distinction points up. Particularly for those whose diagnosis had been delayed and who had pessimized, discovery was described as a "relief." Our data show that a brain tumor was one of the commonly feared alternate diagnoses. Against this possibility, epilepsy seemed less serious. One middle-aged woman trained as a nurse said:

At first I thought it was a brain tumor, so I guess it isn't as bad as that. Well, it was a relief. I mean if you thought you had a brain tumor, wouldn't *you* be relieved to know that it was something as simple as epilepsy, because epilepsy is just not that horrible.

But beyond knowing what it *wasn't*, discovery brings a new kind of order to the experience. To know "what it is," after all, is to see one's experience, both past and future, in a new light. A man who had been in and out of the hospital for various problems involving "blackouts," loss of memory, and depression, said that when he was finally diagnosed as having psychomotor epilepsy,

I was happy. Because I knew what was what. Because for so many years . . . I've had other problems. And my father and mother were there and my father was very relieved and saying, "Now we finally have some answers."* Also, I could [now] write on a job application blank, "epilepsy," instead of "blackouts, with unknown causes."

Although he would come subsequently to see that being able to identify himself as having epilepsy on employment applications was a mixed blessing, he conveys here a sense of appreciation that all of his experiences, correctly or not, can now be represented and summarized by this known medical label.

As we suggested earlier, medical definitions and diagnostic labels bring with them a sense of optimism inherent in the notion of treatment. Conditions for which modern medicine will initially adopt a "hopeless" stance are rare. Moreover, the culture of medicine has as a core proposition the intervention of the doctor toward improving the condition of the patient, or, at minimum, doing no additional harm. One woman, after years of "fainting spells," described her diagnosis as follows:

It was something I could get a handle on . . . what was happening to me and why. I got some medication, which started to control it, and I had a label on what was happening and that was very important to me, because to be having these things happen that nobody knew anything about. It wasn't so much that it was epilepsy but it was something that people knew about at least and could be controlled and I could stop these interminable visits to doctors.

The importance of being "able to get a handle on it," having a name for it, should not be underestimated. Given these and similar comments, we question the medical strategy of substituting "seizure disorder" for epilepsy at the

---

*This parental relief was described by three or four others who told of previous "bad behavior" suddenly being "explained" for parents by the new diagnosis. This was also typically coupled with parental expression of guilt for having punished or disciplined children who, they thought, were being "difficult" or acting out.

time of diagnosis. While the intentions of this change in diagnostic language are to allay stigma and discourage negative historical meanings associated with epilepsy, the phrase "a seizure disorder" may not bring closure to the kind of doubts, anxiety, and searching for "answers" that describe most of the experience in this chapter. One woman spoke directly to this point. She had what she later learned was a grand mal seizure while at work and was taken to the hospital. She said of her doctors:

> They never used the word [epilepsy]. They say I have a "seizure disorder." They don't like using the word "epilepsy" to anybody. I realized I had epilepsy cuz the doctors kept saying, "You've got a seizure disorder and you've gotta take Dilantin," and then [when I would tell others,] people would say, "Isn't that like epilepsy?" And I looked up epilepsy in the dictionary and I saw it was defined as a "seizure disorder." I went back to my doctor and said, "Do I have epilepsy?" and he said, "Well, we don't want to use that word." But for me, using the word . . . literally calmed me down, made me less anxious. Knowing I have something I could call something. I had a disorder I could give a name. *Literally* made me more relaxed. But initially I was terrified. Nobody *told* me anything except to take my medicine.

While we may quibble with Balint's description of diagnosis as bringing order to disordered experience, to know "what I have" is a key turning point in illness experience.

FOUR

The Other Side of Care: Parents and Family Life

One place outside the hospital where illness has been studied is in the family. Over the past two decades, social scientists and others have turned their attention more and more to illness and the family (Davis, 1963; Litman, 1974; Voysey, 1975; Burton, 1975; Featherstone, 1980; Locker, 1981; Speedling, 1982). With few exceptions, however, this research has asked various forms of the following question: What is the impact of illness on the family? This subsumes a number of more specific questions, such as: How do parents manage their

child's illness? What does a child's illness do to relationships between spouses and siblings? How does the illness
of a parent threaten family stability? What kinds of adaptations do family members make to illness? How do parents
and other family members deal with various health care
professionals? While these and similar questions certainly
are important, they almost never lead to related questions
having to do with how the family appears to the person
who is ill. Even when illness and the family have been studied, then, such research tells us little about being ill in a
family. In this chapter we look at the family and illness
from the view of people who themselves have epilepsy.
Not surprisingly, the world of family life, and particularly
the relationships between parents and their children, takes
on a quite different cast.

The view of parents and family life we present here is
of course incomplete. The experiences and events our respondents spoke about are products both of our questions
and agendas and their selective recollections. Moreover,
we should keep in mind that our data are our respondents'
perceptions and recollections of parents, siblings, and
spouses. The other family members' perceptions of relationships and events, of themselves, of what they "actually"
said and did, of how they felt, and so on, would differ from
our data. They would offer another reality and portray different experience. It is just such experience—how children's illnesses look to parents, that has been examined in
the growing body of research mentioned above.

Our data do, however, allow us to address a variety of
questions. We discuss the nature of parent-child relationships as the child's source of information about and interpretations of epilepsy. In particular, we are concerned to
show the importance of parents as arbiters of moral meanings of epilepsy, and how parents can influence children's
understandings of and strategies for managing epilepsy in
ways quite contrary to what they may intend. We give particular attention to the importance of parents' willingness

to talk about their child's epilepsy and to the impact of what they did or did not say. Finally, we address parental "worry" and "protection." Familiar to all parents and children, these become particularly salient and consequential concerns of parents whose children have epilepsy. The "other side" of all these forms of parental care—how they "look" and "feel" to those who are the objects of them— seems to be considerably less sanguine than conventional wisdom suggests.

PARENTS, CHILDREN, AND EPILEPSY

It is a truism that for most children, parents are crucial sources and mediators of experience (cf. Ziegler, 1981). This seems so particularly when children are very young, but only somewhat less so through adolescence. Less acknowledged in the social science literature, yet part of everyday experience, are the ways in which grown children continue to give parental feelings, concerns, and interpretations considerably more than passing attention in guiding their own conduct. The aging mother who says of her adult and similarly aging son or daughter, "He'll (or she'll) always be my baby," acknowledges bonds of influence and attachment that certainly do not end with legal or financial "independence" (itself something of a curious idea). Parents and children typically participate in continuous although shifting patterns of commitment, influence, and dependence throughout their lives. Moreover, parent-child ties are usually what sociologists call "asymmetric," meaning that one person in the relationship takes and is given more power or influence than the other. While it may be true, as some gerontologists have suggested, that adult children and aging parents often in effect exchange roles of authority, the nature of the influence of adult parents on their young children is in general considerably more profound.

One of the most significant ways parents shape children's lives is by making sense of things for them at times when they themselves seem at a loss or are unwilling to do so. It is not an overstatement to say that when we are young, parents or parent-figures interpret the world for us, indeed, even control our access to it and its impact on us. They mediate, inform, translate, shield, expose, and direct us both about what things are and how we might confront and manage them. This is no less true for illness than for other objects and events. It is not surprising then to find our respondents remembered parents as particularly important in how they came to know about and understand epilepsy.

For those who said they were diagnosed during childhood and adolescence, parents were usually the first people to give a name to what they had experienced but did not "understand." Respondents recalled their parents telling them "what it was," or, in the case of diagnosis at birth or during infancy, they recalled parental stories about discovery. The "it" in such accounts typically referred to a seizure or series of seizures, although this word was not then available to them or, in most cases, to their parents. There were many stories of how parents "noticed I was acting funny and took me to the doctor," or how "I passed out and my parents rushed me to the hospital," and so on.

Parents did not always react so quickly, or provide their children with immediate, direct information about epilepsy, seizures, and what was happening to them. Sometimes they delayed this process considerably, stretching it into years in a few cases, before children were given a name and vague explanation for why they had been in and out of doctors' offices and hospitals, had been taking various medicines, and had continued to pass out, "black out," fall down, "feel funny," and "lose control." Not surprisingly, people recalled these prediagnosis events as fearful and anxious. One man who could not remember a time in his life when he was not taking medicine said:

> I always had been, as far as I knew, taking some . . . it
> was like a potion. I didn't know what it was and I
> really didn't bother to ask. I thought, "Well, my par-
> ents know what they are doing." I trusted them. I
> didn't really learn [about epilepsy] until I was six-
> teen. . . . I had a seizure, classified by the doctors as a
> grand mal seizure. That's when I got kinda concerned,
> 'cause I *didn't* know. I got really frightened. Not too
> long after that, mother said, "Well, maybe we should
> go see a neurologist."

It is difficult to imagine what this man and other respondents must have thought when they suddenly lost consciousness and control of their muscles, convulsed, fell to
the ground, and shrieked involuntarily.

A woman diagnosed at age thirteen said her parents refused to discuss what was wrong with her or to talk with
her about her feelings and fears:

> I was a very queer child when I was growing up. I can
> remember going to school. I had this problem, and I
> knew I had this problem, and it was somewhat hard to
> deal with because it was below the surface and I
> really didn't fully understand it. I knew there was
> something amiss but didn't know quite what.

A middle-aged English woman told of a similar parental silence. It lasted a year during a period at about age twelve
when she was having what she later learned were seizures
at school. She said her "conscience was working over-
time," and when she heard her parents talking about a
friend who had schizophrenia and had to be "put in a
home," she thought they were talking about her. She said,
"It had an incredible impression, not knowing [what was
happening to me] for a year." Our respondents explained
such delay and concealment as due in part to their parents
wanting to deny the possibility of a problem, or to mis-
guided protectiveness. Some said perhaps it was because
they themselves were too young: their parents did not
think they could manage it, or wanted to wait until they

were older. Others believed it was more that their parents could not "handle it," delaying in the hope that time might prove what they had discovered about their child to be, after all, not so.

Not all parents practiced such concealment. Some respondents described learning "what was wrong" in a direct, open, and rather immediate way. One woman diagnosed when she was thirteen, said her parents "didn't beat around the bush trying to make it really simple. They just told me that's what I was . . . and it's a disorder of the nervous system. You have a seizure and then you're fine." Another said her parents were open with her about epilepsy "from the minute that I had understanding. I mean, they've always been open." A 28-year-old man, diagnosed as a small child, recalled that his parents said little but approached epilepsy in a "very direct," "very serious" manner: "It was faced in a very direct—the problem was addressed in a very direct manner, you know. There's something physically wrong here and we're gonna do this . . . take these drugs and try to help it." Such a "direct" approach typically portrayed epilepsy as a medical problem, seizures, as a "normal" symptom, and emphasized the importance of following medical regimens, particularly taking the prescribed medication, as *the* way to manage it.

SETTING THE STAGE: OPEN AND CLOSED PARENTAL STYLES

Our respondents' recollections suggest that parents did this interpretive work in quite different ways. Some adopted an open, matter-of-fact definition of epilepsy as a medical problem. Others pursued an almost complete silence and denial that, ironically, told their children whatever epilepsy is, it is "bad"; "something we don't talk about"; even something that pollutes (see M. Douglas, 1963) or spoils the worth of the child him or herself. Barney Glaser and Anselm Strauss (1964) have defined such different styles as open and closed "awareness contexts." These differing parental interpretations appeared, not surprisingly, to be consequential. Children's earliest memories of how parents reacted to their diagnosis seemed to set the stage for how they themselves would interpret epilepsy subsequently. It taught them sometimes harsh lessons about how to manage it as they grew older.

THE OPEN STYLE: EPILEPSY AS A "NORMAL" MEDICAL PROBLEM

Parents who adopted an "open" interpretive style defined epilepsy as first and foremost a medical condition: as something, that, although unfortunate, must be "accepted," managed, taken "in stride." They gave their children basic information about the condition, were willing to talk about it and about how their children felt, and typically counseled a similar style in dealing with others. Respondents whose parents adopted such a style often credited their parents with helping them "deal with it." Epilepsy was, in effect, presented and treated as a "normal" medical problem, with the order and hope this medical frame implies. Such definitions do not trivialize epilepsy or the child's experience. They do, however, portray potential negative effects of epilepsy on one's life as something that can and will be controlled. Epilepsy should be taken into account, its symptoms and effects managed "rationally" according to medical rules and regimens, but not allowed to become something more intrusive. Respondents recounted such parental definitions, often with a sense of appreciation for their subsequent utility. One man said:

> The family and parents of an epileptic child are extremely important as far as I'm concerned. They are the key to the whole ball of wax . . . in recognizing that you have a problem in the family but not let that

control the total actions and the whole livelihood
and the whole future of the family. Accept it and go
on about doing what has to be done to maintain an
even keel.

The themes of maintaining perspective, accepting epilepsy,
and going on with one's routine activities and future plans
were central in recollections of how "open" parents helped
children cope by supplying such minimizing definitions.

Not being treated as special or different made it easier
to take epilepsy as part of one's normal routine. Some said
they learned from their parents that whatever epilepsy
was, it was "not important," meaning not an impediment to
being normal. One young woman of seventeen said she
was able to tell most people she met about her epilepsy.
We asked how she came to be so open about it. She said:

Oh, my dad really helped me a lot. Him and my mom
were the first people that, you know, said, "See, it
really doesn't matter." And he knows about four guys
that work for him that have it and he doesn't really
care. *It's really helped me.*

She added that her father had encouraged her to attend an
Epilepsy Foundation meeting and had also bought her a
medic-alert necklace to wear. A middle-aged man credited
his success at coping with epilepsy to his parents and how
they managed it when he was growing up:

I felt just like a regular kid. I did anything and everything any growing boy would do. [It] was not that
great big a deal because I had very good, intelligent,
understanding parents and this was the key. Perhaps
for a bit I felt like I was a little special, you know,
I've got to take it easy and whatever, but every effort was made not to bring this to the forefront in
my growing up.

Such parental management was seen as carefully intentional. One man, diagnosed at age thirteen said his parents
were sensitive to the potential impact of epilepsy on "a
young person's image":

> They [parents] were very careful about it. In other
> words, whenever they talked about it, it was never
> discussed as something very important. They tried to
> be casual about it as if it were perhaps a terminal
> cold. I think they tried to be careful not to be
> oversolicitous.

They were "careful" *not* to be careful: not to isolate, or set him apart from the typical involvements, participations, and experiences children have.

Parents sometimes told their children that having epilepsy would not limit or restrict what they planned or set out to achieve. One woman said her father assured her at sixteen when she discovered she had epilepsy, "It's not gonna slow you down any. You can still be in gymnastics and do everything else." Aside from the medical wisdom or even accuracy of such advice, pairing minimizing definitions with news of the diagnosis tended to cast epilepsy immediately as less debilitating, less serious. One woman who had severe seizures as an infant but who had been free of them for several years credited her mother and father, but particularly her mother, with helping her cope by refusing to define epilepsy as permanently disabling:

> I think it's the way my parents handled it. Knowing
> what my parents went through . . . and my mother. I
> just can't believe what they went through to save
> me . . . to control it . . . as open as they were and hon-
> est with me. My mother wouldn't go with the answer
> that I was gonna be an epileptic for the rest of my life.
> She did a lot of research . . . she [wouldn't] take no for
> an answer.

Having defined epilepsy as not generally disabling, parents reminded their children they should not be tempted to "use" it as an excuse for poor performance. The woman just quoted said:

> If I came home from school with bad grades, she
> [mother] says, "Now, I don't want you to use this as an
> excuse, because when you were a child you were an

epileptic and now you might have slowness and problems." She said, "You can do it. You might have to
study harder than the next person or your best
friend." She always pushed me to do better.

This theme of "not taking advantage" of epilepsy, of sickness, emerged in a variety of places in our interviews. It
was particularly characteristic of those who adopted an
open, controlling stance toward their condition, and it
reflects precisely the kind of social control of illness that
Parsons (1951) believed necessary to prevent what has
been called the "secondary gain" (Waitzkin and Waterman,
1974) of being ill. Exempted from routine role and general
social obligations, the ill may find the social legitimacy and
effectiveness of medical excuse inviting. Professional medical personnel therefore must periodically warrant such
exemptions.

THE CLOSED STYLE: A ROUTE TO DISABILITY AND DEPENDENCE

These open, minimizing parental interpretations of epilepsy emerged clearly from our interviews. But stories of
parents who had a considerably harder time coping with
their child's condition were much more detailed and told
with great emotion. In fact, the closed, maximizing style of
parental response seemed to be considerably more difficult for the child to manage than the physical aspects of
epilepsy, and its impact is a central theme in our study of
epilepsy and of illness more generally.

Parents who adopted this style were described as
"shocked," "embarrassed," "ashamed," and "fearful" to learn
their child's diagnosis. These reactions spoke volumes of
negative moral meaning to their children, even though,
ironically, in many cases few words about epilepsy were
ever actually spoken. One woman remembered this kind

of reaction to her diagnosis at age fourteen. She said it was
first "disbelief" and then silence:

> Complete disbelief. Y'know . . . "We've never had any-
> thing like that in our family." I can remember that was
> very plainly said almost like I was something, like
> something was wrong. "*We've* never had anything like
> that in our family." They did not believe it. In fact, we
> went to another doctor. And then it was confirmed.
> And so I started takin' medicine. We never talked
> about it again. I just took the medicine. They got it
> refilled and I took it, and never talked about it ever
> again.

Another woman, whose sister also had epilepsy, said her
mother was "ashamed or embarrassed [by it], and the word
was never spoken . . . [and] seizures . . . that word was
never spoken. I forget how she phrased it . . . 'something
you can't see but don't tell anyone.'" We asked her if as a
child she had a sense that epilepsy was something "bad."
She said, "Oh, yes. Definitely."

This sense of parental shock, disbelief, and accompany-
ing silence conveyed a powerful sense of rejection. One
young woman of twenty-two said, "Basically, I think I'm
ashamed [of my epilepsy]. I don't know why I'm ashamed. I
think my mom is embarrassed for me and has made me feel
ashamed." We asked her why she thought her mother felt
that way. Her answer gives insight into the subtlety of
moral meanings contained in talk. She said:

> Oh, like one time we talked and she said, "Oh, I could
> have just died a hundred times for you," or "I could
> have . . . ," you know, because she was upset that this
> [epilepsy] happened to me. It's just something that's
> kept under . . . it's not let out. It's not brought up.

In these and similar reactions as well as in the absence
of talk about epilepsy, parents "told" their children that
epilepsy not only was disabling, but also shameful even
though they may have sensed physical and experiential

evidence to the contrary. The English woman whose parents kept her diagnosis secret for a year said their refusal to talk about it was perhaps the most profoundly consequential thing affecting how she came subsequently to deal with it: "I mean, they, the fact that they had never told me and couldn't cope with me, I felt was a total rejection of a child by that parent." We asked if it would have been easier had they been willing to talk about it with her: "Oh, absolutely, yes. It would, 'cause I'm a person who prefers thrashing stuff out and they're not. They're in that typically English middle class . . . parents who [say] . . . 'It's not nice to talk about those things.'" It became clear to us as we read and reread these interviews that talking about one's fears and concerns, even merely talking about epilepsy as a medical condition that one "has," was an important way of managing, of gaining some sense of "control" over it.

Sometimes parents did talk about epilepsy, but in a way that maximized it even further as a personal disability. This kind of talk took two forms: a catalog of the things one could not do because of epilepsy, and parental coaching for the concealment of epilepsy from others.

Disabling Parental Talk: "You Can't . . ." We call parental talk "disabling" if it sounded the theme of restrictions and detailed the things a person with epilepsy could not hope or expect to do. The specific "don'ts" and "can'ts" varied according to the particular family, its social and economic location, and, to some degree, to the physical realities of the child's seizures and medication. Young men and, most particularly, women were sometimes told they could not hope to marry or have children, and that they may have difficulty forming lasting relationships with members of the opposite sex. One 18-year-old woman described her mother's recent advice: "She seems to think whatever I've got I've inherited . . . and she came out and told me she didn't think I should have kids because of the way [my] uncle [is]." This woman's uncle also has epilepsy.

Boys and young men were also warned about the un-likelihood and problems of marriage. One middle-aged man who had epilepsy since he was a small child, recalled talking with his parents about it. He said: "Oh, yeah . . . that's where I learned that I could never think of getting married." Although he learned later that people with epilepsy could marry, he added, "But I'm so used to keeping myself away from the public . . . I'm too quiet." Another man, diagnosed at age fourteen, said although his parents treated him "differently" as a result of epilepsy, it was difficult to say just how. His wife, present during the interview, added: "Well, it [epilepsy] held you back. They told you you were incapable of doing things." Incapable, unable, not fit, incompetent. These and similar words describe the message conveyed to children by such disabling talk.

Several restrictions were mentioned again and again. "Working around machinery," being "responsible" for others, confronting circumstances of great stress or situations that demanded concentration and alertness, all were defined as impossible. Sometimes forbidden jobs and activities were, in any case, unlikely choices. One man, diagnosed at age eight, said: "We [he and his parents] talked about it some, y'know, when I had seizures. It restricts . . . what you're gonna do later on in life, like you don't want to be a lineman or something like that with epilepsy." We asked him if he had ever considered that kind of occupation. He said he had not.

Many stories about restrictions came from men. Some parents, while thinking epilepsy certainly unfortunate for anyone, seemed to consider it particularly handicapping for sons, given the alleged greater responsibilities they were, as men, expected to carry. One woman bristled with anger when she related a recent conversation with her mother:

As a matter of fact, just the other night I was talking to [my mother], talking about epilepsy . . . and she

said, "Well, you know, it's a terrible thing to say but
it's really better you girls [she and her sister, both
who have epilepsy] came down with it instead of
the boys."

She said she had two brothers and that her mother's attitude "really created a bad atmosphere." A man, diagnosed
at age six, talked about the point in his life when he discovered what epilepsy was, what it meant. He said:

Well, I discovered it when my mother thought to put
a lot of, uh, barriers up there. "Bill, you can't do this,"
"Bill, you can't do that." "Bill, take your pills three
times a day," or, "If you don't take your pills. . . ."
Mother told me I had brain damage . . . [at] about the
age of eight.

He said he was sheltered by his mother: "She gave me too
much loving, which is no good. She'd try to compensate or
something for it. And I believe she overcompensated."

＿Another man diagnosed as a young child said his father
would talk to him about epilepsy: "Mostly he told me I'd
never be able to do things like everybody else could.
Couldn't drive, couldn't swim, couldn't be alone." He
added:

One main thing that really stuck in my head was my
father always told me and my mother too . . . I'd
never be able to live a normal life, y'know, [like] I
couldn't get a job where any tools were around, or
machinery, couldn't drive, couldn't go out climbin'
hills or something. Couldn't be in the boat.

We asked if these were things he had planned on doing as a
child. He said: "I don't know if I wanted to 'til then, but
after I heard that, I wanted to do it! At times I had to prove
to myself I was normal, y'know, I guess. Or, prove to other
people."＿What did he mean by "normal," we asked: "Uh . . .
[that] I could do other things without, y'know, somethin'
happenin'. If I ran around the block I wouldn't have a seizure." He and others said that they, in effect, had to "work"

at being normal in the face of their parent's advice and definitions.

But this work was difficult and the stakes involved were high. Those respondents who were unable or disinclined to resist these parental definitions of epilepsy, quite aside from its physical aspects, were less likely to work at proving to themselves that they were, after all, "just like everybody else."

Coaching for Concealment. Some parents also specifically counselled their children to conceal their illness from others. In doing this they in effect told their children that other people held similar definitions and that all of the limiting predictions about the impact of epilepsy would come true if it was discovered. The only way to prevent this was to keep it as secret as possible. We discuss in Chapter Seven how parents were among the most effective teachers of the stigma of epilepsy. Such cautions and admonitions often came with vague, fearsome allusions.

An 18-year-old woman, noting that her mother kept the diagnosis from her for three years, said:

[She told me] "There's something wrong in your head. Don't ever tell anybody." Yeah, she told me there was something wrong in my brain. I felt like a fruit. . . . I really didn't know what the medicine was for. She'd always say, "Don't ever tell anybody that you're taking pills for anything." She said that they'd put you in a special class, you know, for dummies.

Against the possibility of such consequences, it is not surprising to find that this woman took her mother's advice quite seriously. She said during the three-year period before her diagnosis she told no one and never talked about what was happening to her. When she discovered she had epilepsy she said, "I was smart enough then I knew what it was, but I never had actual seizures where it was obvious and so there was no reason to tell anybody. I figured I'm one of the lucky ones that doesn't have seizures that often, so why should I tell anybody? So, I didn't."—A middle-aged woman who was diagnosed at seventeen said her parents insisted she not tell anyone:

> Couldn't tell a soul. I couldn't tell my grandparents, who lived next door. I couldn't tell my cousins, my best girlfriends. . . . "Just tell 'em that it's your period." They [parents] were ashamed; they thought it was something to hide, so I thought it was something to hide also. I couldn't accept it. I couldn't accept myself, nor could I love myself. . . . It was just hush-hush. —

The price our respondents paid for being coached for such concealment was high. Not only did they have to formulate various strategies to "cover" seizures and epilepsy in public, as well as having to "lie" in a wide variety of situations, including applications for jobs, insurance, and driver's licenses, but they carried the burden of someone whose essential self was flawed or spoiled (Goffman, 1963).

Some women told us how their mothers warned them against telling prospective mates. When we asked one woman if she told her husband about her epilepsy before they were married, she said:

> I talked to Mom about it. She said, "Don't tell him because some people don't understand. He may not understand. That's not something you talk about." I asked her, "Should I talk to him about passing out?" She said, "Never say 'epilepsy.' It's not something we talk about." —

This woman followed her mother's instructions. When we interviewed her she had been married to this man for seventeen years and had kept her secret secure, even though she had seizures regularly and took medication.

Even the interview for this research became a topic for coaching by the mother of a 21-year-old woman. She said that the letter we sent about our study asking her to be interviewed arrived at her parents' house. Her mother opened and read it before her daughter returned home from the university. She told us: "My mom said that she just didn't think it was necessary to talk to anyone about it since it wasn't that serious and she didn't think it was really anyone else's business." She said there was no more discussion about it. We asked her what she would say if her mother asked about the interview: "I'd probably just say I didn't do anything." Not only were these children encouraged to conceal their epilepsy from others, they learned how to conceal more generally. This woman, to avoid a "discussion" about why she agreed to be interviewed against her mother's advice, would simply lie. Aside from whether concealment is wrong or right, it requires us to hold back, cover up our feelings, thoughts, and hence, part of our selves. Such concealment contributes further to the social isolation this closed parental style produces.

Given the foregoing, it is not surprising to find that parents who adopted the closed style conveyed a sometimes profound sense of rejection to their children. They expressed poignantly, through painful words, that there might be "something that was wrong" with them, that they were "imperfect" in their parents' and hence their own eyes. One woman diagnosed at age fourteen said:

> I think my mother would prefer not to know [about it]. She went home and cried [after finding out], which didn't help matters. Things were sort of bad enough on me, but to go home and think you disappointed your parents. That's hard to accept. My dad tried real hard not to think that things had changed . . . and my mom just really did a job on me. She took it real hard. She thought it was a disgrace, really, to have something wrong.

A divorce was credited to epilepsy by a man who said his father "would not accept . . . that there might be something wrong. . . . From what I understand, he just would not accept it." His disappointment did not stem from something his son *did*, but rather because of what he had—because of what *he was*.

One woman told a story of her relationship to her father after being diagnosed at age nine. She wept as she said:

> Dad is the kind of person who was too proud to admit
> something was wrong with his child, and Mother was
> kind of apprehensive; she didn't want to find out any
> bad news. Dad caused a lot of psychological prob-
> lems. He was the type of person who didn't want any-
> body that had something abnormal, and my sisters
> were straight A students. . . . [I think] he didn't think
> as much of me because [of it].

Talk of "perfect" children was offered against the background issue of etiology, of a search for the cause of epilepsy, of "where it came from." Respondents told of over-
hearing parents and having direct conversations with them
about whether or not epilepsy was "in the family." This
often led to discussions of whether or not it could be
"blamed" on one or the other family line. The next question typically was *whose* family was the possible source.
Such concerns often amplified the undesirability of epilepsy when family members attempted to defend their
own genetic heritage with such statements as, "*We've* never
had anything like that in our family!"

Reports of failure to meet parental expectations offer
us an opportunity to point again to the complexity of the
issues involved and the kind of insights, and limitations,
our data allow. We do not know what these parents *actually* said or did to their children. What we do have are recollections of parents by children, most of whom are themselves adults. The views of family life that we portray here
should not be seen as correct or incorrect, nor should the
sense of rejection and imperfection described be credited
to parental action alone. This *sense* of failure is produced
as much by our respondents as by their parents. This is
apparent in one woman's comments that having epilepsy
had "ruined" her goal of being a "perfect daughter." She
told us that this was one of the most difficult things she had
to deal with:

Well, during my whole growing up time I always
wanted to be perfect for my parents. I always wanted
to do everything they wanted—to be their perfect
little girl. That's always what I wanted and it ruined
the picture. I couldn't be perfect anymore because
something was wrong with me. That's the way I felt.

While wanting to be "perfect" emerged from the particular
parent-child relationship, she herself was a *participant*
rather than merely a helpless object of such ideas. The
"victims" of such devaluing meanings unwittingly help to
make them come alive, a point to which we return in the
discussion of epilepsy and stigma in Chapter Seven.

WORRY, PROTECTION, AND
CONTROL

Parents contributed further to their children's sense of
being different, special, and dependent. In stories that
sometimes cut across the open-closed distinction, people
talked about how much their parents "worried" about
them because of their epilepsy, and of how "protective,"
even "overprotective" they were. The more we heard
these stories of how parental worry, care, and protection
looked to those who received them, the more we were im-
pressed by the paradox. It became clear that the love, care,
and attention children with epilepsy received, and that
sick people and sick children in particular receive, have a
darker, less apparent face, one that reveals something not
only about the impact of illness but about the nature of
these "normal" relationships as well (see Ziegler, 1981;
Comaroff and Maguire, 1981).

While virtually all our respondents said that they expected their parents to "worry" and "protect" them "the
way all parents do," they told of chafing repeatedly under
the watchful eye and "worry" of their fathers and, most
particularly, their mothers. In one way or another, our re-

spondents said they took this parental attention into account. Sometimes it weighed very heavily on them.

A sense of this "weight" came most often in response to our question about whether anyone in their family ever had done anything unintentionally to make having epilepsy more difficult to deal with. One young woman diagnosed during childhood said her mother "worried about it and I could sense as a kid that it bothered her, and that bothers me that it bothers her." Another, diagnosed at age twenty-five, said, "[I] had pressure upon me because of me worrying them [parents], causing them problems . . . that if I went someplace they were under a tension until I got back safely."

The things parents worried about varied. Not only were they concerned that their child might be in harm's way, of "What might happen if . . . ," but those who coached concealment also worried about others finding out. One woman who had epilepsy since she was a small child said of her mother:

> Well, I'm sure it aged her because she worries so damn much about people finding out. Well, she worries about her kids all the time; that we weren't home, you know, if we weren't home at a certain time or didn't take our medication, that you were going to have a seizure, or she could be called at work, or somebody would find out. . . . A tremendous amount of worry.

Our respondents saw this "worry," if not a "burden" for their parents, certainly as something that required a good deal of energy and time. Worrying was, in short, grounds for subsequent work that these parents did as part of their parenting.* Parents, and particularly mothers, of children with epilepsy had, it seemed, a good deal of extra work to do.

---

* We appreciate the suggestion that worry can become grounds for work, offered to us by Anselm Strauss.

Virtually everyone who recalled such parental effort said it was and remained distressing to them. Not only was their parents' worry itself a "worry" to them, but such great concern seemed to add more tentativeness and dependence to lives that already had been threatened by these elements. One 19-year-old woman who had had epilepsy since infancy, said her mother worried about her all the time, whether she was in the house, out shopping, or even asleep:

Like, when I go out shopping by myself, my mom worries about me. When I'm home late, my mom worries about me. When I'm taking my bath, my mom pounds on the door, "Are you all right? Are you all right?" you know, to make sure . . . and that bothers me.

Moreover, a parent's worry could become a child's. This woman's mother, through constant concern for her safety and her competence to manage an independent life, had sown doubt in her daughter's mind. Perhaps she did have something to worry about. We asked her about her plans for the future. Did she think she soon would be able to live alone, apart from her parents? She said, with some hesitation, "I would probably drive my parents up the roof, [but] I think I would . . . I think I would probably have to be extra careful, but I think I can." It was indeed an appealing idea, but she had specific reservations:

The only thing that bothers me now is I have my convulsions mostly in my sleep, and I'm afraid of . . . what if I swallow my tongue? What if I can't get out of this, I'll die. And I feel like when my parents try to wake me up and I wouldn't wake up, you know, that would be really scary.

She added, "It scares my mom, but she checks up on me."

Worry and protection are of course believed to be normal elements of parental love and care, indeed, perhaps of all relationships defined in these terms. Our respondents' comments, though, suggest that while some concern, care, and guidance is expected and even desired, too much could become a burden. This worry, particularly within the context of the asymmetric or unequal quality of parent-child ties, easily became control; it could isolate, restrict, and limit. In short, it too could disable and make dependent. Some of the younger people we interviewed talked about the control of worry and protection from very fresh memories. A physically active boy of seventeen recalled how difficult it was for him to abide by his mother's rules that kept him in the house almost constantly during the period just after diagnosis at age ten. He said the undesirable consequences of this protection were all the more clear in the context of his brothers' freedom:

> All my brothers used to come home from school, change clothes real fast and presto, they were gone . . . and they wouldn't come home until supper time. After supper, they was gone again. I used to beg her [mother] to let me go and she said no. And then finally, my uncle said, "Well, God, you can't keep him tied up in the house all the time because he might get worse. You're just givin' him time to sit and think about it." After I started going out I just quit thinkin' about it completely.

The "care," his uncle worried, might be worse than the "disease." His advice to give his nephew less time to "think about it," to "dwell on it," was consistent with much of the folk wisdom about having epilepsy we heard in our interviews. Such protection can limit not only vulnerability, but opportunity and growth as well. The young man continued:

> When they [mother, aunts, and uncles] did stuff like that [imposing restrictions] it just got me madder and I got ornery and that's how come everybody says I'm mean. My brothers say that I'm mean now because they used to keep me in and that just made me worse. Not the sickness . . . because my brothers had been out copin' with problems on the street, and when I

got there the only way I knew how to cope with them was to fight it out . . . instead of talkin' about it.

While this protectiveness may have given him a convenient explanation for his "meanness," he portrayed it as making things more rather than less difficult to manage.

Some respondents said that they adapted eventually to such protection by seeking isolation. One woman, diagnosed at age nine, framed it in terms of being treated "different," kept from various activities and involvements. She said that her "whole family . . . always did treat me different. They always were watching out for everything I did. Just like I didn't hardly go anywhere. I didn't do much of anything because everybody was always being careful: 'Don't do this. Don't do that.' It got to a point where I just didn't wanna do anything."

They said it was as though they were "children," or "little children" for whom others, and particularly parents, had still to "watch out" and "take care," being themselves unable to manage the decisions and events of everyday life. This view was expressed with considerably more chagrin by those who as adults had to contend with such treatment. One 27-year-old woman said her family had always "tried to treat me like a little kid . . . that's about the worst you can do." This concern was conveyed in recollections of parents who tried to "baby" their children as a result of epilepsy. One woman said:

> They tried to baby me. I think they wanted me to live with them the rest of my life. They still do. They still treat me like I'm ten years old. They come up to my place and tell me how to take care of my kids, and how to do this and how to do that. . . . They don't think I can take care of the kids.

Another woman, thirty-five, who had had epilepsy since she was nineteen, said she thought her relationship with her parents had been affected by her illness:

> Oh, I think it would be better if I moved to a different

town and was completely away from them. They kind
of treat you like you are still real young. They live
[here]. They think they still have to be very protective. They give a lot of advice.

These and similar comments suggest the complication illness adds to the already imbalanced quality of parent-child
relationships. Epilepsy, and any illness or disability, can become good grounds on which parents can presume that
this dependency will be extended beyond adolescence.
Parents often see themselves as having a kind of open-
ended responsibility for their children and what happens
to them. In consequence, what might be typical or routine
parental concern is heightened and becomes, unwittingly,
a device for sometimes highly restrictive control.

In addition to shielding children from possibly hurtful
and distressing experiences, parents sometimes tried to
withhold various kinds of information that they felt would
only be upsetting or disturbing. One 33-year-old man told
how his parents kept from him the fact that his brother had
been involved in a serious car accident. When he found
out, he said:

At that point, I went through the roof. I explained
very bluntly everything else that I wanted to know.
Something like that went on and I wanted to know
about it right now. They proceeded to inform me that,
well, they "didn't want to upset me." And I said, "By
Goddamn, you're gonna get me a hell of a lot more
upset by *not* tellin' me than if you do."

It was the fact that his parents had made these decisions
for him that was so distressing. Usurping the prerogative
and the experience to know about such things not only
placed him in a position of dependence on his parents, but
also told him that, in their judgment, he simply could not
handle the emotional stress.

On balance, it seemed that parents' desire and attempts
to help actually magnified the significance of epilepsy for
our respondents. The more their time together was spent

on epilepsy, medication, seizures, precautions, instructions, reminders, and the like, the less time there was for other topics and activities. As one 35-year-old woman said of her well-intentioned parents, "They are always trying to help too much." She said they had actually made coping with epilepsy more difficult:

> Like, they don't let you forget you have it. If they
> could only just forget about it, you know? I think they
> are very well-intentioned, but it's just that it's always
> in the back of their mind. "Well, you have epilepsy
> and I'll do this for you and I'll do that for you."

The experience of always having someone willing to do for you can become disabling in that when others do for us, we do not or are not as likely to do for ourselves. As the young man who said he had a "tough" reputation put it about his mother and relatives, "They just wanted to watch me, take care of me, and I hated that. I hated it with a passion 'cuz I like to be left alone, to do things for myself." To "do things for myself," to be independent to make choices and decisions within a context of love and support, was what many respondents said they wanted in relationships with parents, family, and others.

The significance of this independence or space to become a full-fledged, competent person is apparent in those few cases where it was allowed to develop. Not all parents were remembered as restrictive in their love and care. Some respondents spoke of parents who were "wonderful about it," "just great," and who, in effect, provided both the minimizing interpretations discussed above and the freedom from isolating worry and protection. Parents remembered as not "anxious," "worried," or "overly protective" were recalled as being of great help in coping with epilepsy. One man, in response to a question of whether or not his parents had been protective of him as a child and youth, said:

> Never. My parents encouraged me to do anything that
> I felt I was up to. They never said, you know, they of

course said, "Never . . . don't play in traffic," but they
never said, "Don't do this" or "We don't think you
should do that, it's too exerting for you." In fact, they
advocated that I try out for whatever I thought I was
up to. And to do the best I could do in whatever I
tried out for, whether it be scholastically or physically.
My parents have been wonderful about it all through
my life.

Aside from what this man actually did pursue, his comments suggest that he had a sense that the decision was his
to make, that he could choose and try what he liked, without his parents worrying and protecting him. A young
woman diagnosed at age twelve said that her parents "never
restricted" her:

Maybe they felt that if they restricted me that it
would be psychologically damaging for me because
like, you know, if I couldn't go swimming, couldn't
do this, you know, after a while anybody who is restricted is going to feel weird after a while, you know,
abnormal.

But parents found it difficult to follow what may have been
their own best inclinations. And in the face of cultural definitions of the relationships between the ill or handicapped
and the well, and the overwhelming readiness to "help,"
our respondents found it difficult to resist such parental
help without risking the relationship itself. Many said they
did not like this help and advice, but most seemed to toler-
ate it, even as adults.

FIVE
Seizures and Self

Illness is a humbling experience, a great leveler. It reminds us that despite social position and personal accomplishment, talent or charm, we rely on the trouble-free operation of our bodies as a taken-for-granted medium through which we create and express our selves.

Although we continue to learn new things about the connections between body and mind, the operation of our bodies is defined in general to be quite beyond our willful control. Hearts continue or fail to continue pumping blood, neurons transmit electrochemical impulses, tissues grow, develop, and die quite independent of our intentions.*

---

*Suicide is, of course, the obvious exception. In addition, we can and often do contribute unwittingly to this process through our lifestyles and habits. Such techniques as "biofeedback" and the "relaxation

This becomes only too apparent to us (for usually it is not) when we become sick. While such changes may not actually represent a "loss" of control (since we never had it in the first place), the incapacity and limitations they often bring render our experience, daily rounds, and in some cases, future plans, quite changed.

In this chapter we discuss seizures as an instance of involuntary body changes that may obliterate one's sense of self control and contact with the world. They are abrupt reminders that self does depend on body. We look at seizures through the eyes of those who have them, discuss the kinds of problems they present, and describe how people cope. The experience is summarized accurately as one of "assault," and the reaction, as one of "struggle."

HAVING A SEIZURE: LOSING CONTROL

When we asked people to tell us what it was like to have a seizure, many found it difficult to answer. A few at first said they did not know what a seizure is like because they did not "experience" it. One man said:

One thing that you're probably going to find out in interviewing epileptics is an epileptic doesn't know what an epileptic seizure is. That, I think, is one of the things that's of most interest. I have never seen an epileptic seizure so I don't know what it is from the outside. To me an epileptic seizure is those symptoms that I feel before the seizure. And you've heard a million of these: kind of vertigo and losing consciousness and fighting to maintain your consciousness, then finally waking up and finding out that actually you did have a seizure . . . and just disorientation that you feel

---

response," while providing detail about these mind-body connections do not seriously challenge the dominant view.

and the stiffness of the muscles and the teeth that have chewed the gums and the whole shmear of things. To me this is an epileptic seizure, but I've never seen one.

This description is typical of people's responses. They would talk about what they were doing or how they felt just prior to losing consciousness, and then describe the feelings and perceptions when consciousness returned. Our respondents called seizures "black outs," "blank spells," and spoke more generally of the experience as like "being away." One man answered another who taunted him about his bizarre behavior during a seizure by saying, angrily, "Look, buddy, I don't know what happened. I wasn't there."

Not "being there," people often called on witnesses, usually family members or friends, to document and describe their seizures. When we asked how often he had petit mal episodes, one young man said, "Well, I used to have them all the time, I guess. But Mom is the one that tells me, 'I haven't seen one on you for a year.'" A student, living away from his family, said he "didn't know" how frequently he had "little seizures" because "there's no way of telling besides being around other people." A junior high school student told a story of how a friend called her at home to tell her she had had a grand mal seizure at school. She thought she had gotten sick and was sent home. Her reaction was disbelief and shock that she could have had a seizure without knowing or recalling it.

Some said they knew what their seizures were like as a result of witnessing someone else's. These observations became the basis for imagining their own seizures. One man told of witnessing a seizure while having physical therapy in a hospital: "I was shocked, but yet I'm glad I saw it, because now I know what other people perceive if I should have one . . . and how they might act or react." A woman told of her reaction to a dramatization of a seizure she and her husband saw on television: "It's horrible. I saw it on TV once and my husband said that's exactly the way it happens. I really couldn't believe I could do something like that."

Those who did offer descriptions usually drew on the analogies provided by their physicians. A common one was that seizures were "like an electrical storm in the brain" or that they occurred "when electrical circuits get out of control." One man said his physician told him seizures were "like a room full of mousetraps" into which one might throw a ping pong ball. The ball then sets off a "chain reaction" and all the mousetraps are sprung. Another described seizures optimistically, as something "natural" and "interesting," rather than "terrible":

It's the body's automatic self-preservation mechanism. I mean it does that to release that tension . . . it's like a very dramatic example of tension and then release. It's why after, say, a grand mal seizure, there's always a period of very deep sleep. It's just the body rejuvenating itself. To me it's a fascinating and very optimistic thought. I think that kind of approach can help people understand it as something natural, not something aberrant.

This normalizes seizures as part of the body's "wisdom" (see Cannon, 1932). It portrays them as miraculous "natural" events typical of the health-maintaining processes common to all bodies. Such definition, as this man himself points out, can become a resource in the work of coping with and attempting to control the impact of seizures, something we discuss more in the next chapter.

Whether or not people experience seizures, all our respondents agreed that usually they were frightening and in some cases "terrifying" events. This fear was not primarily of physical injuries from a fall or other seizure-related accident, though such injuries were familiar to many. And while the metaphor of physical assault or attack was used often to describe the experience, such as "like being knocked out" or "hit on the head with a hammer," it was not the body they saw as most under siege. Rather, and most importantly, seizures were experienced as a threat to, a suspension—indeed, the absence—of the social person, the self.

Our respondents talked a good deal about losing control of body movements and consciousness. One woman said: "I suppose anything you don't have control over is really pretty scary. Specially when your body's concerned. I think that scares a lot of people . . . not having control over what your body does, especially when you don't want it to do it." Another, who described herself as a victim of a "force outside my power, my control," spoke directly to what was so fearful about such events. We asked her how she felt about seizures:

> How do I feel about seizures? I feel very painful about them. It's a process of total disintegration of one's whole self. I lose control. I have absolutely no chance of being able to do anything about it. I feel a victim of a force outside my power, my control. It does affect the self image 'cuz you are . . . you're helpless in the hands of something.

These and similar comments remind us how intimate is the connection of body and self, and specifically, how much the latter depends on the unproblematic operation of the former. When our bodies are threatened, then, so too are our selves. Sociologist Erving Goffman (1963) has described this threat as particularly notable for afflictions of the face and voice. Seizures variously impair the capacities of both as ways to offer a conventional presentation of self.

Some respondents recalled the feelings of losing touch with the physical world: "It's one of the most horrifying experiences in the world. I feel completely disattached from my surroundings . . . floating off someplace." Another said, "It was the weirdest feeling. Like I wasn't in my body." One woman talked about "something" that she tried to "keep at bay": "It's a feeling of something that begins to crowd out

the external perceptions. Like that other world was crowd-
ing out what is there . . . and you're trying to keep at bay
whatever it is that is trying to press in."

For others, seizures occurred without warning. Descriptions were of the type, "One minute I was . . . and the
next thing I knew, I had had a seizure." A young man recalled how one night he got out of bed, went to the bath-
room, and the next thing he could remember "was getting
wheeled on a wheelchair in the hospital. It shook me up. I
thought, 'What's goin' on here?'" A woman described a seizure she had while shopping: "I remember standing there,
I was buying a bra and I remember giving the woman the
bra and my charge plate . . . and I don't remember another
thing until I was home." Seizures were for some so sudden
and memory obliterating that they developed what could
be called formulas or rules of thumb to help them decide
what had happened. One woman said she used the vision
of an emergency room with medical personnel over her as
a sure indication she had had another seizure. Others spoke
of waking up to find themselves on the ground or floor
with people staring down, asking, "Are you all right?" and
saying "Don't worry, we've called an ambulance." For those
with petit mal or absence-type seizures involving momentary lapses of consciousness, clues came often in the sudden realization that "no one was talking and everyone was
staring at me." For those whose seizures occurred typically
in their sleep, a sore or swollen tongue or mouth, produced by jaw contractions characteristic of grand mal seizures, was the confirming evidence. Feelings of "complete
exhaustion" and having "wet the bed" told others they had
had a seizure during the night.

Many descriptions of seizures seemed almost surreal
or fantastic: being "helpless in the hands of something,"
"overwhelmed," "hit on the head," "out of control," and
"floating off someplace." Respondents were reticent in giving these descriptions. Sometimes, having said them, they

would add the disclaimer, "I know that sounds strange, but . . ." or "It sounds weird, but . . ." Given these images and descriptions, we perhaps can appreciate more some of the historical definitions of epilepsy discussed in Chapter Two. How would we have made sense of such events and descriptions outside the context of today's medical and scientific knowledge?

SEIZURES AS SOCIAL EVENTS: TROUBLE FOR OTHERS

The perceptions of what it "feels like" to have a seizure have a counterpart in how people believe seizures appear to and affect others. Rarely are seizures completely private events. Someone else is usually present. Most people said that they had had at least one seizure in public; all said that they had "worried" about it. As we turn our attention from the "interior" experience of seizures to their significance for those who witness them, we turn to the perception of seizures as social events. The problem of "lost control" remains central, but in considering perceptions of others' reactions, we begin to understand how the meaning of seizures is constructed and where the control that is "lost" comes to reside. We discuss this social face of seizures under the themes of embarrassment, the creation of medical emergencies, and the distribution of responsibility in social settings.

EMBARRASSMENT

Our respondents described seizures as embarrassing events. "Whatever else," writes Goffman (1956: 264–265), "embarrassment has to do with the figure the individual cuts before others felt to be present at the time." This is, of course, true of all social affect, such as guilt, shame, and even pride (Garfinkel, 1967: 38). These feelings emerge in us as a consequence of defining our own conduct in terms of the moral contours of the setting. Embarrassment, in particular, is our response to the perception that we have failed to meet others' expectations, and that these others have recognized this.

Just how "embarrassing" seizures were depended on how visible and public they were. Virtually none who had only nocturnal seizures described them as embarrassing.* Similarly, seizures that were brief, momentary lapses of consciousness ("absence" type), were less likely to be called embarrassing than the grand mal type. Such seizures often were quite easily concealed, even in ongoing social interaction. This was, however, contingent on the situation and on who else was involved. A college professor, for example, told of having a "light" but "embarrassing" seizure while presenting an important lecture; a salesman described a "little" seizure as "difficult" when it occurred "right in the middle of my presentation to some clients"; and a young woman said she was "embarrassed" due to a "blank spell" she had during a coffee break with a few neighborhood friends who did not know of her epilepsy. Particularly for those who adopted a highly secretive strategy, even "little" seizures could become embarrassing for what they might reveal.

For those whose seizures were not easily concealed, the sense of having violated social expectations was considerably stronger. As with certain other kinds of embarrassment, this feeling comes from a sense of having interrupted or disrupted what others are doing. It sometimes also comes from becoming the center of others' attention. One man described such seizures by saying, "Everything stops." Those others who have stopped then turned their

---

* Occasionally, these people would say they were sorry or felt guilty if such events disturbed family members, but "embarrassing" is a word not found in such descriptions.

attention to him. Goffman (1956: 266) described the embarrassed individual as "present with . . . others, but . . . not 'in play.' The others may be forced to stop and turn their attention to the impediment."

Impediment is a particularly good word to describe how people felt in such situations. "It's not only the embarrassment that I feel," said one man, "it's the fact that it's an imposition on anyone around me." Another told of how he had a seizure in church during the minister's sermon: "I just interfered with . . . all at once, everybody's looking at me. Everything brings attention to me when I do have one of them in public." And one woman described what she called a "very difficult" seizure while dining with her husband and friends at a business-related banquet. She described the scene upon regaining consciousness: "When I came around, there's people all around and everybody's interrupted what they're doing. They'd stopped everything. It was just horrible, just awful." This woman commented more generally on others' reactions: "People draw their attention to you. People look at you, stand around and peer at you. 'What's goin' on over there?' I hate it. I just really hate it."

Beyond being disrupted, our respondents believed others were usually frightened by seizures, particularly, as it was put, "if they don't know what they are." Not knowing what they are means not identifying them as symptoms of a medical condition. The most dramatic reactions came from naïve others who were close friends or family. Respondents perceived that, without the ordering frame of medical diagnosis, others were at a loss for making sense of what they saw. One woman described the reaction of her sister-in-law during a holiday visit:

> my brother and sister-in-law and I . . . they'd just married and he'd obviously not told her about my seizures. I had a seizure in the middle of the night. I mean, she was absolutely scared out of her wits. She

didn't know what to make of it. She was screaming and hysterical, saying "Why? What does it mean?" One man described a seizure he had while in a "compromising position" with his "first true love": "We were in the front seat of the car one night and I had a seizure right on top of her and she didn't know what the hell was going on. Just scared the living hell out of her." Some even said to witness a seizure without "knowing what it is" was worse than having one: "They're more painful for the people seeing me than for myself, because I'm unconscious."

Besides being embarrassed, people said they felt guilty, remorseful, and responsible for intruding on and frightening others. This felt imposition varied according to the intimacy of the relationship and the particular setting. It was not a reaction limited to situations involving strangers. People expressed similar feelings when seizures disrupted or inconvenienced family members and close friends. One man said that he seemed always to have a grand mal seizure during family Christmas celebrations. He said, "I really screwed it up bad. I wanted to come back out and show them I can act right." Another said he wanted to tell people, "I'm sorry it happened, that I upset the dishes or I broke this or wrecked a good party or whatever. I'm sorry. Remorse, failure, this type of thing."

Having said this, however, people seemed to feel that "wise" witnesses to seizures—those who defined what they saw as a normal symptom of the medical condition epilepsy—were less likely to react with fear and rejection. This reduced their own feelings of embarrassment, guilt, and shame. Such wisdom came from both previous experience and education. One woman, whose daughter also had epilepsy, said of the latter's seizures: "I'd had a little more experience with my own by then" and it was not so frightening. Another described her mother's and sister's reaction to her public seizures as "good": "They're cool," and "like normal as soon as I come totally to." A man said he told his supervisor and fellow employees if he had a seizure at work, they should "just leave me alone and I'll be perfectly all right." He said such seizures had occurred and "everything was fine."

The ideal reaction from others is, in effect, to "take it in stride" and, at all costs, not to overreact. A woman told of how easily things went when she had a seizure at a job in a typing pool where others knew of her epilepsy: "I was typing and I just stopped typing . . . yet none of them do anything about it. They just continue typing and just for a few seconds I stop and then I continue typing too." If people felt they could have a seizure around others who would define it as routine, they themselves would feel little embarrassment. Such reactions were most common in close relationships that offered an insulating cushion of shared biography against which the seizure took on minor significance. A woman said about others' reactions:

> Mostly it's having a seizure happen with people I know very well and so they tend to have a sense of who I am. I'm sure it would be different if I walked into a shopping mall and had a seizure there. I'm sure people would have difficulty responding to that. But mostly it's been in relationship to people who know me well and know that's part of who I am.

Another woman grew up living with her grandmother who had regular and sometimes violent seizures. She said: "They became 'normal' because I saw so many; that was just something that grandma did."

This is another instance of how redefinition moves something problematic, even threatening, to the new status of something to be expected. When respondents described having seizures "as a part of who I am," and urged others to regard them as such, they embraced a definition of themselves as "a person with the medical disorder of epilepsy." Thereafter they could use this definition or identity to "make sense" of their experience both for themselves and for others (see Lemert, 1951).

"CALL AN AMBULANCE":
SEIZURES AS MEDICAL
EMERGENCIES

Naïve others, when confronted by a "bad"—usually meaning grand mal—seizure, seemed to think something was very seriously wrong with the afflicted person. A sudden shriek or cry, unconsciousness, a fall, violent muscle contractions, drooling and sometimes incontinence; such images are the raw material from which naïve witnesses apparently defined seizures as life-threatening medical emergencies. In modern society, when people suddenly act this way, and particularly when we do not have normalizing or neutralizing definitions available, we call an ambulance or medically trained personnel to intervene.

Respondents said that naïve witnesses to their seizures thought they might be dying. One man described a particularly dramatic reaction of a close but unknowing friend with whom he was traveling abroad. Both had just taken the drug LSD when the seizure occurred. He said:

> The guy thought I died. We were very close and had been through a lot. It really blew him away. It just had an enormous impact on him . . . just an incredible fear. He told me that when it first happened, all he could do was run around the room . . . because he didn't know what to do.

Another young man quoted his friends after a public grand mal seizure. They said, "Boy, you should have seen it. You turned purple and blue, and we thought you were dying." And a middle-aged woman recalled her young son's reaction at seeing one of her first seizures. Her neighbor told her later that the young boy came running to them, crying, "Come quick, Mom's dyin', Mom's dyin'."

In the absence of wise "interpreters," naïve witnesses reacted by calling an ambulance. They defined what was happening as a medical emergency. One woman commented with some empathy on how others reacted to a public seizure she had while walking through an alley in the city: "I'm sure it was pretty frightening. A woman found me and just screamed and then a policeman came and they got the ambulance and took me to the hospital." One man summarized others' typical reactions to his seizures: "A lot of times I end up in hospital because . . . folks have been frightened into calling the ambulance."

For those accustomed to having seizures in public places, this reaction is often more troubling than the seizure itself. Those who minimized the significance of their seizures said they would much prefer simply to be left alone to "get my bearings" and go on their way. Naïve witnesses insisted on defining such events as medical emergencies, even against the individual's protests. A woman offered a particularly elaborate example of this collective definition when she had a seizure on a trans-Atlantic flight approaching a major eastern city:

> It was as if the whole airport had been geared up for my arrival, with police and ambulances . . . it was extraordinary. There was a wheelchair at the bottom of the steps, police helped me off. There was no customs, no passports, nothing. My luggage was extracted from somewhere magic. The two guys sitting next to me on the plane said, "How are you getting back?" I didn't know them from Adam. I said, "I'm going to take the airport bus." They said, "Oh, no, we'll take you." By the time I got home my roommate said, "Are you all right?" I said, "What do you mean?" She said, "Oh, I just had a call from the airport authorities." I felt very embarrassed about the whole thing. I wanted to shrink out of sight about it.

Even in their "helpful" reactions, others made her seizure something much more than it was, at least in her view. By defining it as an emergency, others took control of and directed its unfolding. The woman, apparently overwhelmed by these reactions, went or was taken along, thus validating the emergency definition. She would have preferred it otherwise. She called it the "most embarrassing" seizure she ever had. Such stories, tell us that during seizures people "lose control" not only over their bodies, but over subsequent definitions of what is going on, who they are, and what should be done to and/or for them. It appears that others are quite willing to temporarily assume this control and quickly place the afflicted person in medical hands.

One woman had a seizure while shopping in a large department store. She said:

> I was not aware that it was coming on. I was just . . . walking towards the door and just went down. And they took me to the hospital, y'know, and I just kept saying, "I'm fine, I'm fine." I'd come around then and they wouldn't let me get up. I think the store was afraid of liability or something. I kept saying, "I'm fine, just let me up," but they insisted.

Once she got to the hospital emergency room and was checked by a physician, she turned around and went home. Another woman spoke about this "overreaction":

> I was just walking down the street and I had a blackout and people get so upset. They call the ambulance. Right away they take it into their own hands. "Well, she's had a heart attack," or, "She's diabetic." This one man brought me inside and I was just telling him it was nothing and he said, "Oh, just wait" and he called the ambulance and they all hold onto you real tight, you know? They won't let you go. They all think there is something really wrong with you and you're trying to get away from it. "I have epilepsy," I told them, but they still think, "Well, you have to go to the doctor first, ambulance." And, you know, the ambulance costs twenty some dollars.

Many complained about this unnecessary cost. Most said, in effect, "It's just something that happens to me." Once at the hospital emergency room, medical personnel usually validated this definition. After being "checked over," they were released and told to go home. The woman quoted above said when she arrived at the hospital, "I just told them, 'Well, it's just epilepsy I have and you can't do anything.' They said, 'Well, okay,' so I finally took the bus home."

Some became angry at others' ignorance. One woman turned to epilepsy volunteer work as a result of her frustration and anger at others' reactions to a seizure she had had. She recalled:

Everybody was around me . . . pointing, hysterical. The company nurse was there . . . the guard from downstairs was there with a wheelchair. They wanted to take me to the health . . . and I got so mad . . . at their ignorance. That's exactly when I started doing volunteer work. I said, "There's nothing wrong with me. . . . I'm okay. I feel a little sleepy right now. You don't have to bring me to a doctor. If you'll let me lie down for half an hour I'll be okay." And they wanted me to leave.

The disparity between the individual's and others' definitions of the situation was a familiar theme in our conversations about public seizures.

These recollections were part of a larger perception of others' reactions to seizures as "overblown," "extreme," and, in fact, difficult to deal with. One man said the way others react immediately after a seizure, when the person is regaining consciousness, "is the most crucial time in an epileptic's life." In particular, he pointed out that well-meaning others, by barraging the individual with questions at a time when the person finds it difficult to respond, actually intensify the impact of the seizure.

The people that come up to a recovering epileptic and say, "Gee whiz, how do you feel, how do you feel? Are you all right? What'd you have for dinner? Do you remember going to school today? Do you recall all this stuff? How about it, huh?" You want to answer every question they can pose to you, to show them you're all right and you want to communicate that ev-

erything's great with me . . . and you can't even say
your name. You can't tell whether it's dark or light or
even what dinner is. Just let the epileptic alone, let
him go, he's not going to hurt himself. Come back in
twenty minutes and have a cup of coffee or whatever,
but just leave him alone. I have been frustrated to the
point where I get extremely angry.

When asked later if he thought others sometimes exacerbate the impact of a seizure by their reactions, he said,
"Absolutely, and I think most anybody that has epileptic
seizures or any other kind of seizures would feel the
same way."

Through their reactions others can unwittingly reinforce negative definitions of epilepsy and of the people
who have it. One woman recalled that a high school class-
mate sometimes had seizures. She described them as "traumatic" for herself and other students and told of how "the
teacher would run back and use the tongue depressor. . . ."
A young man said his high school coach "cleared the locker
room" when he thought this young man was going to have
a seizure. Such reactions by others contribute to the definition of seizures as fearful emergencies. This definition,
though often at odds with the individual's own perceptions, becomes the dominant or public framework through
which the situation is defined.

SEIZURES, RESPONSIBILITY, AND SOCIAL COMPETENCE

When naïve others are confronted by a seizure and define it as a medical emergency, an important shift occurs in
the distribution of social responsibility. The "work" of
carrying on interaction is suddenly stopped, new definitions of the situation are made, and a reorganized division
of labor emerges in which those at hand take on new responsibilities, new "control" that resided earlier with the
afflicted. We believe this occurs not just with seizures, but

with illness more generally as it affects social interaction and relationships. The shift suggests that a moral view of illness, distinct from deviance (Parsons, 1951; Freidson, 1970) and stigma (Goffman, 1963), becomes relevant. While the medically ill may not be blamed for their condition, and perhaps not even devalued, their illness can become the basis for others having to do more "work," and take on more and sometimes heavy responsibilities. This tips even further already unbalanced relationships and heightens the ill person's dependence on others. Not only do they suffer the physical assault of the seizure and the moral weight of stigma, but they become "risks," "liabilities," and "worries" in others' eyes, a point well documented in our earlier discussion of parental care.

Witnesses to seizures, and particularly the naïve, have a frightening responsibility thrust upon them. Before them is a person behaving in a bizarre fashion, convulsing, unconscious, having difficulty breathing. Respondents said these witnesses "feel uncomfortable" because usually they "don't know what to do." To "do nothing" in such situations is counterintuitive (even relatives and close friends had to *learn* to "do nothing"). It also requires serious account-giving later on. Most people said that others found this responsibility heavy and unwanted. One woman said of others:

> I think they panic. More than anything else, it's the idea "I don't want to be around you if you have one 'cuz I don't know what to do." I think I can say that about a neighbor guy. I think he's like my husband. As long as sickness is over there, fine and dandy . . . even if it's someone getting sick to their stomach. "Just stay over there because I don't know what to do with you if you are sick."

She added that as far as her friends are concerned, they think "I'm fine, as long as I don't have one [a seizure] in front of them."

This woman's likening of seizures and sickness is instructive. Earlier in the interview, she had offered the same interpretation, saying that as a child she learned, "If you are sick, go in the corner and come out when you're feeling better." Two underlying social assumptions emerge in her comments—that the "sick" should be segregated and that "well" others must bear responsibility for them. The "sick" are seen to have a legitimate claim on the available and relevant "well" to help, give aid, or, at minimum, bind up the social wounds illness often brings. Such expectations are particularly strong when the "well" and "sick" are face to face.* Thus, while illness and responsibility officially are channeled through the relationship of physician and patient, lay persons around the ill also share this culturally defined obligation.

When people had seizures in public places, they assumed others should "know what to do," or that they would do "whatever is necessary" to prevent undue harm, injury, or even death. Whether this first aid might consist of making small talk to soothe and cheer, moving the person to safety or rearranging the physical environment to prevent injury, rolling the person on the side to facilitate breathing, or calling or not calling medical authorities, our respondents believed that they had a legitimate claim on the presumably well to "be responsible" since they themselves could not. This shift of responsibility, however, could come at a high price, measured in terms of the person's competence in others' eyes. Having called for help—by dint of having a seizure—respondents often found others thereafter "never quite the same."

Employers and work supervisors were mentioned often. If they had been called upon to "take over" during past seizures, respondents believed them to be wary, suspicious, and watchful. Those who had had seizures became

---

* For a preliminary and conceptual view of such relationships within the family, see Corbin and Strauss (1982).

people who could not be "counted on" to handle routine situations. One man told how he had tried to return to work after a severe head injury from a fall due to a seizure at work:

> When I tried to go back to work, we played all kind of hell trying to get me back. My doctor said I was ready physically, able to go back to work. The company insisted I go see their doctor. He said, "What did your doctor say?" I told him and he says, "I don't know what the hell you're doin' here then." I says, "I don't either." Finally, they said, "Okay, you can come back to work next week." Then they put it off for another week. The typical excuse was they couldn't decide back in the main office. Then, when I came back they wanted me to wear my hardhat . . . in the office! My boss . . . my immediate supervisor . . . I don't think he really understood the whole thing. Pure ignorance on his part.

This man had the feeling "they were keeping an eye on me" for almost two years after he returned to work full time. Even then, his full responsibilities—traveling through the state as a technical expert—were restricted because his supervisors feared it "might be too much" for him. Another man had had a grand mal seizure while clerking in a department store. Although he was kept on, "I was under strict limitations. I could do just this and so, and if I stepped out of line there was a directive that it could mean termination." And finally, a woman told of a kind of surreptitious surveillance by her coworkers after she had had a seizure at work:

> Like after I fall on the job, I've got people coming up and checking on me all night to see if I'm okay. You get to feel like a little baby after a while and you don't get treated the same. Every once in a while you'll see somebody coming in like to go to the bathroom on my floor when there's one on their floor, or the guard

comes up and he says, "Hummm, I thought I smelled
smoke up here." In a way it makes you feel kind of
bad you can't operate on your own two feet.

This woman and other respondents felt that after a seizure
at work, others did not fully trust them. "It's almost as if,"
one woman said, "they were expecting me to have another
seizure."

Such questions about one's competence were not limited to work situations. The issue of "risk," however,
seemed most common in organizational settings, including
schools and rehabilitation programs. In what must be the
ultimate irony, one man told of being banned from a vocational rehabilitation program because he had a seizure
while at the program workshop:

They asked me what I wanted to do. At the time I had
a cane, so I said, "I wanna refinish it." So, I had some
stripper in a great big pan and I tripped and fell, face
forward, into the stripper and passed out. So they said,
"Well, he had a seizure." But I don't think I did. I in-
gested so much of that stuff into my system . . . I don't
think it was a seizure. But they kicked me out and
told me I couldn't come back. I said, "Man, I thought
that's what you guys were here for." He says, "Well,
we can't have you on our property as long as there's a
possibility of you having a seizure, because you could
sue the state."

He had become, due to his "seizure," a liability to an organization dedicated to removing precisely such limiting
definitions of people with epilepsy. These rehabilitation
people, using what they themselves were committed officially to diminish, proved to this man that as long as he
had seizures, he was just too much of a risk to be given
responsibility.

Respondents often used the words "risk" and "responsibility" to describe how others perceived them. Driver's
license and insurance restrictions were mentioned often.
Of all problems associated with epilepsy, driving restric-

tions were one of the most troublesome. A driver's license and access to a car have become insignia of full social competence in our society. Beyond this symbolic significance, restrictions increased our respondents' sense of dependence on others. While many relied on public transportation, these people said they rarely participated in social activities because they either could not get to meetings and events or felt uncomfortable about "always relying on other people." When they rode with others, their schedules were determined by the drivers.

Insurance restrictions against people with epilepsy opt them out of another taken-for-granted social participation and protection. Life and health insurance is difficult to obtain. Insurance also was a reason employers gave for why it was "necessary" to "let you go" from jobs after a seizure. People were told, "we just can't afford the risk of your having an accident, hurting yourself and someone else."

People with epilepsy who have public seizures often see themselves in others' reactions as tentative, uncertain, unable—as, in short, someone who cannot be counted on. Even when others know what is happening, namely, an epileptic seizure, they may move the individual into a category of "people to be watched" and "cared for." Such reactions from others, or, more accurately, the perceptions that others react in this way, contribute to the definition of self as dependent. People who have seizures, indeed, people who are "sick," are set apart from the "well" and typically are placed under the latter's care. This segregation occurs both physically and symbolically, as people find themselves impaired not only in body but also in the ability to assume and carry through normal responsibilities. Given the potential social and personal impact public seizures can have, it is not surprising to find that our respondents devoted a good deal of attention to ways to prevent or at least mollify this threat. In the next chapter, we examine their strategies toward this end.

SIX

Controlling Seizures, Protecting Face

Seizures, like illness more generally, are things to be minimized, controlled, and if possible, eliminated altogether. They are fraught with negative potentially discrediting meanings about the self. When others witness their seizures, people feel embarrassed, humiliated, and anxious about others' subsequent treatment and definitions of them. As a result, those who have had public seizures try hard to minimize their impact.

TOWARD REGAINING CONTROL: SEIZURE THEORIES AND PREVENTIVE WORK

People who have seizures must contend with an unknown yet constant degree of uncertainty in their lives. This uncertainty most respondents incorporated into the planning and pursuit of their daily activities. They could never be sure that a seizure would not suddenly incapacitate them. We asked one young man, for example, whether he thought he still had epilepsy even though he had gone a year without a grand mal seizure. He said: "I think it's like that atomic waste that they bury. You never know if for some reason an earthquake will come along and work it right back out of the ground, or if it's gonna stay in one place." One woman said she had never had a grand mal seizure, but that she was "still afraid of 'em": "I've never had one, but it's there. It's like lurking back there . . . yes, I may have one. Each time I've had a medication change it's scared me . . . you know, that it would start up something."* This uncertainty was particularly difficult to manage in situations where a seizure would bring great embarrassment or danger. A young mother described how she felt about seizures by saying, "I think mostly, just frightened. Just not knowing if it was going to happen when I was driving the car with both of the kids or . . . walking across the street. . . ." Another said, "The whole time I was pregnant I kept thinking, 'My God, what would happen if I was in delivery and all of a sudden have a seizure?'" And a man who was a sales representative for a large company

---

*Interestingly, this woman's descriptions of her seizures sound very similar to the clinical description of grand mal episodes. She maintained throughout the interview, however, that she had never had a grand mal seizure, and expressed a great deal of anxiety about the possibility that she might.

said, "I have a fear of, let's say, giving a presentation, for instance, and having an epileptic fit. I am afraid of this. That is a bigger fear to me than falling into a lawn mower or anything else. I think of the public humiliation." This same man later said he believed seizures "bring death a lot closer." As a result of "knowing any minute you could have a seizure, I've rather accepted that. I've got everything all in order."

In response to this uncertainty, people tried to create order and certainty (cf. Hewitt and Hall, 1973). One strategy was to make this tentativeness itself something of a routine. People developed their own theories or explanations for the incidence of seizures. While respondents credited physicians with explanations of "what seizures are," rarely did these professional explanations suffice as guides for understanding their own experiences. The "theories" our respondents developed are an attempt to exert some degree of control by creating a sense of retroactive and prospective understanding of their own seizure biographies.*

In considering such lay explanations, it is important not to judge them by scientific criteria. Their primary importance is the symbolic and practical significance for their authors. They represent first and foremost an attempt to cope with seizures by, in effect, "owning them"—by making them products of one's own cause-and-effect propositions as they are founded upon lived experience (propositions which, incidently, appear to be held even against,

---

* By invoking the prerogative to define their own experience, people display an important kind of social control that operates independently, albeit sometimes parallel to, the official, professional theories of medical science. As Dingwall (1976) and others have suggested, in order to develop a more complete understanding of how people experience illness, we must turn attention to how these lay theories are created, the nature of their logic, and how they articulate or do not articulate with those of the professional medical world (see Locker, 1981).

and perhaps primarily in the face of, professional skepticism). These theories both define and order a set of experiences to which only their authors are privy. At the very least, such explanations render the fearful, unfamiliar, and uncontrollable ever so slightly under control. Beyond that, they often become grounds for preventive strategies.

SEIZURE THEORIES

When we want to develop general explanations of problematic events, we first search for patterns in these events that cut across different situations and conditions. This search for patterns of conduct and occurrence is the basis for inductive generalization or reasoning, whether one is a scientist or layperson. Our respondents often described how they had searched for patterns in past seizures by trying to reconstruct what they were doing just before the seizures occurred. One man's wife said, "We wracked our brains, thinkin', 'What did he do?'" that might have "brought on" this or that seizure. Another woman said she "kept a diary for five years trying to find some kind of relation." She admitted, with some frustration: "I can't find anything. No patterns at all." Those unable to find such patterns were less likely to profess their own understandings over those of their doctors. They were also were less convinced that they themselves could do anything about having seizures, beyond following medical regimen. By transferring responsibility for their condition to medical experts, these people more often embraced the definition of themselves as objects variously at the mercy of their bodies and the "forces" inside them.

Most of the patterns people saw in their seizures were understood as products of following medical "dos" and "don'ts." For example, things believed to precipitate a seizure were fatigue, lack of proper sleep and diet, the absence of generally "healthy habits," a chaotic daily schedule, excessive emotional stress, and failure to take their medication as prescribed. Using these assumptions, some respondents concluded that seizures were products of their own excessive or "foolish" conduct. One man said:

> I don't worry about them, but I very seldom have them. I maybe have one a year and when I do it's usually from me working too hard, not getting enough sleep over a period of three or four months. It's usually my own fault. I try to do more than I should.

This man suggests, as did others, that he has a standard against which he judges how much is "too much" for him to do. Both before and after a seizure, people often referred to "overdoing" as a cause.

This proposition of excess-as-cause is part of the perception of seizures and epilepsy as disorders that emanate from "nerves," the nervous system, the brain, and emotions more generally. Although none of our respondents professed an understanding of neurology, most said they knew they had seen a neurologist and had had EEGs or brain scans. They believed that epilepsy and seizures came from some malfunction "in my head." This vague understanding provides grounds for a "lay neurology" in which worrying about having a seizure could cause one. This worry hypothesis is illustrated in one woman's comments about a recent seizure:

> Maybe I brought it on myself because I was worrying about it. Therefore, if you worry that it's gonna happen, then it's gonna happen . . . like, if I didn't worry about it, then it wouldn't've happened, or probably wouldn't've.

According to this view, controlling worry about seizures can reduce or prevent them. One woman said: "The psychology tied up with epilepsy . . . is very, very strong. You can say what you like about that, but I'm convinced they're related."

For many, worrying about having a seizure was more

troublesome than the seizure. This was true particularly where the consequences could be great. A sales representative told how he thought worry could produce a seizure:

> I'd get in a waiting room and I'd sit there and think, you know, all these people sitting here, "What would happen if I had a seizure?" I'm going to mess up this whole thing. I'd almost talk myself into it because I not only had the feeling of being nervous, but the more I thought about it, the more I talked to myself about it. . . . I started to feel guilty, I started to feel embarrassed, I started to feel all these things like I knew it was going to happen . . . and sometimes it did.

Extending this logic, he reasoned, "If I can talk myself into them, I ought to be able to talk myself out of them." His physician encouraged this proposition. It was tested often and believed by many.

Avoiding situations that made people "very nervous," such as "being out in a crowd," "meeting new people," and "getting up in front of a group," was one strategy. Public performances, sometimes involving no more than carrying on a conversation, were also threatening. Such situations, usually of little concern to "normals," were full of anxiety for some respondents. At the same time, many said stress is a normal part of life. To manage seizures by avoiding stress would require social withdrawal, making achievement of a conventional personal identity all the more difficult. Some said that isolation and idleness could bring on seizures: "They're [seizures] more likely if I'm not doing anything . . . if I'm sitting around too much in one place." Another said, "time on my hands" could almost certainly "bring one on."

Another way people managed uncertainty was to admit and then reject seizures as grounds for concern: "There's no need worrying about having a seizure, because you can't do anything about it anyway." According to this view, seizures "come when they want," in spite of preventive effort. In fact, such effort is seen as a waste of time and energy. Uncertainty is thus turned upside down: it is made certain; seizures become largely unavoidable. Control is achieved by proceeding as if one were indeed normal. One man said he "dreaded" having seizures, but did not "worry" because he could not do anything about it. "If it's going to come, it's going to come. Nothing can stop it." A woman who was a stockbroker said:

> There's nothing I can do. I have a high tension job. I put in very long hours. My social life can be tension creating. I don't want to quit my social life, I don't want to die. I wanna see friends, I wanna see guys. There's nothing much to do. I just try to get some extra sleep.

And another, when asked if she tries to avoid seizures by avoiding stress, said: "No, it's not something that I think about in planning. I don't take it into account."

Our respondents not only had explanations for their seizures, they also often tested them against experience. One young man, a student, said, "I was thinking . . . if I drank a lot of soda again like I did before the last seizure, or study a long time, I might have another seizure . . . you know, where you really get your mind kind of fried out." By generalizing what he was doing just prior to his first seizure (he had yet to have a second), he hypothesized that that kind of conduct might have produced it.* While he was skeptical such an explanation would prove correct, he said he was careful to avoid similar situations, "because I start worrying that it will happen again." One woman, who had earlier mentioned strain and tension as probable causes, added that, on the other hand, she had had seizures at times when she was rested and relaxed. A man who described himself as an alcoholic said he at one time thought

---

* If we free ourselves from the criterion of logical validity in such cause-effect assumptions, however, and consider how this reasoning is useful to, has meaning for, those who create it, we can appreciate more fully the importance of such theorizing.

his seizures were alcoholic convulsions. He subsequently rejected that notion on the grounds that they persisted when he was not drinking. Finally, a woman told how she had formulated and then rejected a hypothesis that "running water" may have caused her seizures:

> For a while I thought it was water, 'cuz I'd go in and turn on, like, for my bath water and . . . the steam would come up and I'd automatically just have one of these feelings. And then I'd go in and flip the kitchen sink on and just . . . running water. So I thought maybe it was just something screwy in my metabolism and I just couldn't handle the sound of running water. But then it would happen out mowin' the lawn or drivin' the car, so . . .

In these and similar instances, people develop "plausible-to-me" explanation for their seizures, first by searching out patterns, making note of antecedent circumstances or situations, then formulating and testing hypotheses to account for the events. While social scientists tend to describe common-sense explanations as unsystematic and uncritical, these data suggest that we should pay more close attention not only to lay theories, but to the processes through which they are constructed, tested, and (like scientific theories) modified in the face of evidence.

PREVENTIVE WORK

The most common preventive strategy for seizures was to take the medication prescribed by one's physician. In "high risk" situations, such as those discussed above, some said they took "extra" medication "just in case." The perceived effectiveness of this varied, but most remained committed to taking medication as a general strategy, often as a "hedge" against the possibility of having a seizure.

Few, however, relied solely on medication to prevent seizures. They used their own experiences and understandings as a source of alternatives. Most of these reflected the "nerves" or "worry" hypotheses, and included various forms of meditation, mind control, biofeedback, self control, and, when possible, avoidance of high risk situations.

One woman said she used transcendental meditation to help control her seizures. She said it definitely helped her relax: "My blood pressure dropped, so I went off the medication for a while and then I went back on . . . because the blood pressure went up." A man said, "I think if I could become good enough at that meditation, and could get into a systematic program of learning exactly how to focus, I might be able to relieve myself of the burden of some of the medication." He said when he felt an aura or warning he used meditation to reverse the seizure. He described the experience as

> battlin' as hard as I can . . . just tryin' to overcome it. I really want to have control over it. If I can get myself relaxed and get my breathing regulated and get my concentration focused, I can overcome that breaking point, that threshold, whatever it is, that turns on the switch, you know, that makes me have a seizure.

One woman became involved in a "mind control" program that produced "fantastic" results and reduced the incidence of both seizures and auras. As a result, she "cut back one Dilantin a day":

> It's a cross between self-hypnosis and transcendental meditation. Since I've taken that course I've not even had an aura. I mean not just the attacks, but I used to have at least four or five auras a week if nothing else. I haven't had one of those since I've taken this mind control thing.

While most had not turned to such organized programs of meditative control, the notion of "getting myself relaxed," "calmed down," "concentrating on not having it," were steps people commonly took to stave off a seizure. Expressing a corollary to the worry hypothesis, many said they believed they could "talk themselves out of" at least some of their seizures. When she felt the sensations of an aura, one woman said she kept her "senses very tight, together. I fight against it, like when you are going to vomit. I say to myself, 'God, I've got to stop this.'" Another man said he used a lot of "psychology" to "pull myself out of them":

> I use a lot of reverse psychology. I have to tell myself things that I should believe that I usually will not believe. I have to tell myself, "I can pull out of this, I can pull out of this. It's not gonna continue." It usually works.

While most were not sure they could actually control the occurrence of seizures, they believed they could reduce their likelihood by remaining as calm as possible.

Finally, one woman described her involvement in a nationally organized vitamin supplement program: "Since I got into this, I've cut my medication down to one Dilantin and one phenobarbitol a day. I was tired of taking so much medication and decided I was going to give it a try." She had had one seizure since starting this program: "I tried to go off my medication completely, and I couldn't do it with just the vitamins."

Others said they adopted general preventive tactics such as avoiding stressful situations or excessive fatigue. Getting extra sleep, reducing alcohol intake, maintaining a regular schedule, trying to keep one's temper and staying out of arguments were mentioned commonly as personal policies. One woman said when she became overtired or overstressed:

> I will really remove myself from the situation that could possibly cause me to have a seizure. Then I'll withdraw to an area by myself and involve myself with something very simple, very relaxing. Listen to music, read a book, lie down. I generally won't drive during those times, and so on. I take extra medication . . . that's about the sum total of what I can do.

Still others took more specific steps, such as avoiding sugar and eating a lot of starches. "Sometimes," said one man, "I get up and walk around"; a woman said she "puts her head down" when she feels as though she is going to have a seizure. "I slap myself in the face," said another, "It usually brings me right out of it." There was a variety of such specific home remedies to reduce the chances of having a seizure.

A quite different approach was to overcompensate. This involved an attempt at what might be called "supercontrol" in high risk situations. The goal of this strategy was to be completely "in charge." One woman told of using this approach as a college student. Confronted with the anxiety of classroom performance in which she could become flustered, anxious, and subsequently have a seizure, she said she spent hours memorizing material. "It was an automatic thing. Like some kind of machine, like I would push a button and there would come this answer." She preferred classes where "there was more limited discussion, like biology class where you were required to have very precise answers." Another man said when he finds himself in situations where he might become anxious, such as chairing a meeting, the "first thing I do" is take medication; the second is to "overcompensate." "I try to maintain control at all times. If I lose control of the situation I have grave difficulty." We asked him how he managed to maintain such control:

> Well, let's say for instance I'm conducting a meeting. I don't let a meeting float around. To me, the floating is akin to the vertigo or whatever you want to call the threshold, long or short as it might be before an epileptic fit. I get a correlation here. Things start to float around, meaninglessness, that type of thing.

Was a seizure more likely under such circumstances?, we asked: "Oh, yes, there's no question about it." He admitted, however, he had never actually had a seizure in such a situation.

All of these preventive strategies were used in an attempt to gain greater control over seizures as "uncon-

trollable" events. Quite aside from the logical or scientific
validity and effectiveness of such ideas and actions, they
order experience and provide some sense of control over
the physiological tyranny that seizures represent. These
strategies are part of epilepsy not found in standard medical discussions.

SOME LINES OF DEFENSE

Beyond general preventive work, people developed
defenses for when seizures did occur. These were adopted
both as a matter of course and as a specific response to
warnings that a seizure was imminent. Both strategies seek
to defend or protect, either by giving attention to others'
potential reactions, or, as emergency measures, to prevent
injury.

ANTICIPATORY DEFENSES

One defense against seizures was to tell others about
them in advance. This included direct disclosure of epilepsy, provision of educational information about seizures,
and instruction about "what to do" should a seizure occur.
Those who used this strategy wanted to reduce the negative impact of seizures on others. "About the only thing
you can do," said one woman, "is to tell people. The more
you talk about it, the more relaxed people become and
then it won't scare them so." Such telling was sometimes
deemed a "responsibility" to others. This sense of obligation comes from how people believe seizures affect others.
If others "know" what they are seeing, they are less likely
to be fearful, and consequently, less likely to feel discom-
fort, or if they do, less likely to blame the afflicted for it.
Warning others about one's seizures, then, was a kind of
self defense.

Respondents felt that giving instructions for what to do
when a seizure occurs lightened the witnesses' burden.

One common direction was "just leave me alone." This usually was elaborated somewhat by suggestions that the observer could move sharp or hard objects, turn the person on his or her side to facilitate breathing, and resist the urge to call an ambulance, depending on the particulars of the event. Convinced that others are both generally and specifically ignorant about epilepsy and seizures, respondents were often more concerned to tell others what *not* to do. Second only to not calling an ambulance was the instruction not to put anything in the person's mouth: "I'm not going to swallow my tongue," one man said. We heard a variety of stories about how well-intentioned bystanders had their hands and fingers bitten when trying to rescue what they thought was an imperiled tongue. In preparing others to witness seizures, our respondents were careful not to contribute to the definition of them as emergencies. We heard often the themes of "nothing much to do," "just let me be," "don't worry," and "do nothing."

Another defense strategy was to wear or carry some form of medical identification—typically, a "MedicAlert" tag or card. Most, however, expressed skepticism about its effectiveness. One man said about a card in his wallet, "I've never had anyone look at it when I had a seizure." Such devices seem to be poor substitutes for direct disclosure and instruction in that once others are in a position to search for cards or tags, the seizure may well be over. Almost everyone said they "should" carry such identification, but few actually did. "I simply haven't gotten around to it"; "I did once, but lost it and didn't replace it"; "I keep forgetting to go in and buy one," were typical responses. Since few saw their seizures as medical emergencies, such medic-alert identification perhaps seemed inappropriate.

Self-imposed social isolation and restricted participation were other ways people defended against the shame and embarrassment of a public seizure. One man said his reaction to the possibility of having seizures was "social withdrawal." Some spoke of their desire not to return to

school after having a seizure. One woman, having the responsibilities of chaperone and driver for her children, yet
legally prohibited from driving because of her seizures,
said she developed a set of "special routes" and "rules."
These kept her off heavily-traveled major streets, out of
rush-hour traffic, and off the road at night. Another, in a
similar situation, said she "drives very little" and "only
when necessary." When she must drive on the highway, she
said she tries to encourage her children to come along, and
"plays games and sings" with them "just to keep my mind
off what I'm doing." With a certain degree of humor, a college professor told of how she dealt with what she called
"sleep seizures" while lecturing: she stood near an over-
stuffed chair so that her fall would be cushioned and mini-
mally disturbing to her students.

A third defensive tactic was to plan to be with a friend
or family member who "knows what to do." These others
serve as body and self guards who can be counted on to
take charge in case of a seizure. The essence of such protective work was typically definitional and interpretive.
One man told of how he himself served this role for a
woman friend when they were dining in a public restaurant:

This girl . . . I take her out once in a while. One time I
took her to the hotel and she had one of them. She
was shakin' there at the table and knocking stuff off. I
took her out in the lobby and sat her there. That's
what I'd want. I wouldn't want to be sittin' there at
the table after coming out of it and having everybody
stare at me. Get away from the crowd. I told them if I
could get her somewheres temporarily, away from the
crowd, I said she'd be all right. Don't need the rescue
squad. I went back in and explained to them just what
the deal was, and to see about the mess. They were
glad to find out about it because they never knew
really what to do to help a person.

By placing himself between the unconscious person and
naïve others, this man was able to mollify embarrassment,

avoid unnecessary "emergency" definitions, and make sense for others of what had happened. As a result, the experience was made considerably easier for this woman.* One woman said her husband once noticed her "acting funny" while they were in church. Before the seizure occurred, he took her outside to their car. When she regained consciousness, he said, "when I noticed you chewing, I knew I had to get you out of there." And a middle-aged man said when he is out in public with his parents, they "watch out for me" in case "I start acting strange."

EMERGENCY MEASURES

When general plans of prevention and various anticipatory tactics fail and a seizure seems imminent, people resorted to a final line of defense. We call these emergency measures because they are initiated just prior to losing consciousness, in response to feelings described as warnings or auras. Their use depends on how accurately people read these sensations as indicators of seizures. Accurate readings, however, were often difficult to make. Experience quite literally seemed to be the best teacher. Even with a history of several seizures, some said they could not recognize auras until after the seizure occurred. One young man said: "It makes me mad that I don't recognize the feeling. If I knew ahead of time a seizure was coming it wouldn't scare me one bit to do any of this stuff . . . to drive, to get my pilot's license, or anything else." Another man said when he first began to have seizures he did not drive much, "because I hadn't learned yet to recognize the signs." As his skill improved, he allowed himself more unrestricted activity, convinced that should a seizure occur he would have sufficient time to avoid anything that might prove dangerous. By contrast, a woman said her lack of ability to

---

* We interviewed this woman for our study. She spontaneously told of this same event and said how thankful she was that the man, quoted above, was with her.

recognize an aura or warning "is why I don't get a driver's license, because I have no chance to take defensive action."

From these and similar comments, it became clear that even when people experience warnings they often do not have seizures; at other times, seizures occur with "no warning at all." Sometimes the auras before grand mal and absence type seizures were undistinguishable, increasing problems of interpretation. One man said: "I can't tell if it's going to be a grand mal or just stay as a strange feeling. I had one driving the car and I stopped down at the corner and just waited, because I didn't know which way it was going to go." "Of all the auras I have," said another man, "only about 5 percent end in seizures." While a few said they had become, as one woman put it, "stubborn," and went on with their business in spite of these feelings (thinking, "it will pass"), most dealt with such uncertainty by assuming a seizure was imminent, took appropriate protective or defensive action, and then "waited to see."

Our respondents often sought "safe places" when they thought a seizure was coming. Quickly lying down or sitting on the floor or in a chair, and steadying oneself against a building were ways to reduce possible injury from a fall. Depending on the interval between warning and unconsciousness, as well as the kind of seizure, people described more extensive last-minute defenses, such as seeking the privacy of some unused room, a public restroom, empty hallway, or even, in one case, a closet. These emergency strategies served two purposes. Beyond reducing chances of physical injury, they were intended to gain privacy. One woman said that when she is shopping or away from home and experiences an aura, she tries to go to her car. She added, "I don't care for an audience." "I try to get away from everybody," said one man. A woman described how she would escape to a nearby restroom while at work and "sit on the floor in one of the stalls" to prepare herself for a seizure.

Safe places can be crucially important for those who keep their epilepsy secret. This same woman described how once, when she felt a seizure coming on, she took cover in the nearest private place, which happened to be a *men's* restroom. She explained, "It was better than out in the hall." Such escape is sometimes facilitated by what one woman called a "reconnaissance"—scrutinizing routine settings for safe places to which she could flee (cf. Davis, 1973). How adequate the cover such places provide depends on how open or closed about epilepsy people are (cf. Glaser and Strauss, 1964). In open awareness contexts, a quiet corner often served the purpose, although privacy was usually preferred. For those more secretive, safe places were harder to find.

Some said they have only a moment or two after an aura before a seizure occurs. For them, elaborate protective and evacuation plans are out of the question. Reflecting the feelings of fear discussed earlier, many said they would simply cry out to whomever is near, "I am going to have a seizure," or, would ask people to hold or shake their hand. One woman said, "I know I am going away from you and I want you to hold me here."

AFTER A SEIZURE:
ATTENDING TO FACE

Once a seizure has occurred, strategies of prevention and defense become irrelevant. Instead, the problem is to assess and deal with damage to face, to one's reputation as a conventional, competent person. In these situations, people try to patch up, smooth over, and minimize, such discredit. In this final section, we discuss how this is done.

One way people tried to contain what they saw as a spreading stain was to draw on the power of "medical excuse." Social scientists know very little about what others actually think about such excuses. From the viewpoint of those who offer them, however, medical excuses are a culturally available and acceptable means of legitimizing sickness as grounds for exemption from responsibilities.

Some said, for example, that after having a seizure in front of others they simply told them that they have epilepsy, that what happened was an epileptic seizure, and that in a few moments they would be fine. Such accounts were given regularly to ambulance and hospital emergency room personnel, both in an attempt to order the situation for these people and to minimize undue problems for themselves. Other respondents said they attempted to explain their seizure to witnesses, "so they wouldn't think I was weird or something." One woman said she thought it better others know she was having an epileptic seizure than for them to think "it was something worse, like being drunk or on drugs." In perhaps an attempt to appear even more blame-free, some told others after a seizure, "I take my medication regularly" but "sometimes it just doesn't work."

This power of medical excuse is, however, limited and conditional. Given the official restrictions against people with epilepsy, such accounting can reap negative and unintended consequences. For example, a man recalled an automobile accident one rainy night. Fearing penalty, he discarded the several cans of beer in his car into a nearby ravine before police arrived. He decided to explain the accident by saying he had a seizure, even though he had not, thinking he would not be penalized or blamed. Much to his chagrin, he said:

> I went home and the next morning a knock came on the door. They said, "We want your driver's license." I said "What for?" They said, "You had an epileptic seizure and ran into a telephone pole. You have to go two years without a seizure before you can have your license back." So, at that point, I moved to another state.

Although free of blame for the accident, this man could hardly be said to be "free." While the sick are not held re-

sponsible for being sick, they are often variously disen-
franchised allegedly for their own and society's good.

Several men told stories of how they and others had
used humor about seizures as a way of coping. These stories
were drawn particularly from people's school experience.
For instance, sometimes one's knowing friends would joke
about seizures, as one man said, to put him at ease and
"make light of it." Most said they went along with such jok-
ing, even though it made them uncomfortable. Fearing to
show affront or embarrassment that they believed would
signal the real and usually great significance they attached
to such events, these men laughed with their friends about
their seizures. One said:

> Well, my friends with their sense of humor started
> telling me all of these things I do while I was in a
> seizure. There were a few obscene things they were
> telling me and they thought that was funny. I suppose
> in their way, they thought, "Well, we'll just make a
> joke of it and then he won't care," which I suppose
> was the best way to handle it. Well, I'd laugh too, but
> I didn't think it was very funny, but you really haven't
> got a choice. I felt serious, but acted the old mask,
> "Yeah, it was funny, wasn't it?" That happened to me
> several times.

Another described a particularly difficult adolescence with
epilepsy. We asked how he managed seizures in front of his
peers. He said:

> The adjustment at that time was one of downplaying
> it because of my fear of being ostracized for it. I re-
> member one friend saying, "Hey, you were foamin' at
> the mouth and everything." I go, "Yeah? Really? Wow."
> That kind of thing, as if it were something "neat." That
> was the only handle I could allow myself to take. I
> mean, inside, you know, I was havin' kind of cardiac
> arrest. I just felt sweat streaming down my bones a lot
> of the time.

Such defenses, although they may have succeeded in terms

of outward appearance, very likely had associated costs in the form of increased isolation. In addition, such strategies of carefully constructed humor likely fooled few of those involved on either side of the experience.

Another fascinating strategy of saving face was to construct definitions of what had happened as something other than an epileptic seizure. This was, not surprisingly, much more common among those who saw epilepsy as a serious moral flaw or who had a great deal of anxiety about being discovered. Sometimes people tried to act as though nothing had happened. This was used primarily by those who had absence rather than grand mal seizures. Some said they never mentioned such "light" seizures to others because that would draw attention to something others may have missed. One man said when he is talking with someone at work and has such a seizure, "I just ignore it." We asked how he answers the question "What's wrong?" He said, "I've never had anyone ask me." Another told of how he once offered covering accounts, such as, "Oh, I'm just tired," and so on. He gave this up, however, because, as he put it, "It just wasn't worth the energy." He admitted such attempts rarely worked anyway.

More typically, however, respondents felt they had to offer others some kind of explanation for their seizures, even when they were only brief lapses of consciousness. Certain that these events were highly visible, they believed that to say nothing would leave others' suspicions unattended. In lieu of this, various "covers" were offered to portray unusual conduct as due to something other than epilepsy.

Covers were variously easy or difficult to construct depending on the movements, sounds, and settings involved. Often, particularly when with friends or family in public, covers were constructed collectively. People would enlist the assistance of "wise" others (Goffman, 1963) who would "play along" or actually aid in constructing such non-epilepsy definitions for the benefit of naïve witnesses. Re-

sources available to individuals and the particulars of seizure and setting increased or limited the range of plausible
stories offered. The perceived plausibility of such accounts
—here and elsewhere—is very important. Clearly inappropriate stories could produce as much or more skepticism about the individual's normal status as saying, "It was
an epileptic seizure." As one young man said after having a
seizure in his junior high school, "The thing I thought most
about was, 'What kind of excuse can I make up?'"

These covering accounts are variously elaborate, from
a simple "Nothing," when asked, "What's wrong?" to complex explanations. One complex scheme was described by
a woman who was a pharmacist:

> At this point I can pretty well cover myself up be-
> cause now when I come out of one I know I had it.
> Like I'll be talking to someone and I'll turn around
> and walk a couple of steps and then I come out of it
> and I'll look back and know they're there and I was
> talking to them, so I'll cover myself up by picking up a
> piece of paper or something or grabbing a pen, like I
> forgot something I was doing before I started talking
> to you.

She said of this strategy: "It may sound stupid, but I think it
works, and it doesn't seem to bother them at all." This
same woman described another example of covering in
which she drew on the artifacts of her work: "Yesterday I
was arguing with a doctor on the phone and I had one. I
knew I had one and what I did after was explain to him that
I was checking the pharmacy literature, covering myself
up. He accepted that fine." She explained that the print in
the books she uses is very small and "it's easy to lose your
place." Since she had reviewed this literature earlier, she
had the information ready to provide when she "returned"
to the phone.

Another said she had a "whole drawer full of excuses"
to cover her seizures. Once she had bitten her tongue severely during a seizure and had difficulty speaking dis-

tinctly. When friends called on the telephone, she would say she had "fever blisters," or she would respond "I bit my tongue, could I call you back?" Other accounts, such as "I have been under a lot of pressure lately," "I'm very tired," "Oh, I'm sorry, I was preoccupied," were used commonly to normalize minor seizures. Such stories sometimes were effective even for grand mal seizures. One woman told witnesses what they had seen was a product of her other maladies, which included heart disease, low blood pressure, anemia and "nerves." She was sure others believed her.

Wise companions sometimes participated actively in managing a definition of the person as normal. One woman's husband helps her cover:

> He covers up for me when I have blackouts. Like in playing cards. If I lay a card down and it's the wrong time or something, he'll make a joke about it. He'll say, "My, you're really getting nervous about this card game, aren't you?" Everybody laughs, but I know what he's doing.

By defining such putatively unconventional conduct as a "fluff," a "mistake," "just not thinking," this woman and her husband construct a normal definition that comes to stand over against possible alternative definitions from unorganized others. Research in the sociology of deviance offers examples of coalitions of family and friends protecting insiders from negative definitions by such neutralizing and normalizing. We know from the work of Erving Goffman (1959, 1963) and Harold Garfinkel (1967) that others can play a crucial role in the drama of impression management. By drawing on this projected and shared definition of her as normal, this woman and her husband used the same kind of definitional process typically applied to people with epilepsy by the larger community. The success of such work varies, of course, according to the plausibility of the covering definition, the situation, the conduct, and the identities of those involved.

SEVEN

The Problem of Stigma: Managing Information

Illness describes a moral condition. To be sick or to have a disorder is to go through something unfortunate, "bad," or undesirable. But the metaphor of illness (cf. Sontag, 1978) further conveys irregularity, victimization, pity, and even revulsion. This moral component of illness is most apparent in the chronic conditions in which distinctions between disease or disorder and self become blurred. A passing cold, flu, or even a more serious acute condition or malfunction do not have the implications for self or identity that chronic conditions do.

Epilepsy, of course, is just such a disorder. As such, it describes an undesirable moral condition. But having epilepsy exposes people to moral experiences considerably more complex than this common undesirability of illness. Specifically, it carries at least two other kinds of morally negative meaning. We have just described a second moral aspect of having epilepsy: what it is like to have seizures and to contend with others' reactions. The sights, sounds, and movements of seizures are analogous to what sociologists call deviant behavior, although this analogy is only somewhat enlightening.* The comments in the previous chapters tell us that having seizures presents a special set of moral dilemmas to those involved.

There is a third consideration that makes epilepsy even more morally complex. It follows directly but is distinguishable from the visual facts of seizures as *the* signifying feature of this condition. It is the stigma historically associated with the diagnosis, the name itself. Epilepsy is a stigmatized illness. We have described some of the predominant elements of these negative meanings and how they have changed while continuing to persist in general form over the centuries. Virtually all of the myths and theories about epilepsy, its causes, and cures reviewed in Chapter Two focus on seizures. Our respondents, almost without exception, treated seizures and epilepsy as closely linked. Yet seizures and epilepsy are distinguishable as objects of social meaning. Our respondents did in fact make these distinctions. It is to the term "epilepsy" that stigma has come to be attached, quite aside from the grounds for this connection. In Chapter Two we discussed the historical and social disrepute of epilepsy. In this chapter, we examine how people experience and deal with stigma in their

---

* Seizures might be called unconventional conduct, although strictly speaking, the movements and sounds involved cannot be considered conduct at all.

daily lives. We comment on the particular kind of stigma people with epilepsy face, the importance of the stigmatized person's perception in the activation of stigma, ways people try to control discrediting information about themselves to mollify the stigma of epilepsy, and finally, how people sometimes use disclosure of epilepsy *as a medical problem* toward this same end.

STIGMA AND EPILEPSY

The most insightful analysis of stigma available is Erving Goffman's (1963) book bearing that title. His opening words are particularly relevant here:

> The Greeks . . . originated the term *stigma* to refer to bodily signs designed to expose something unusual or bad about the moral status of the . . . [individual]. The signs were cut or burnt into the body and advertised that the bearer was . . . a blemished person, ritually polluted, to be avoided, especially in public places.
>
> Later, in Christian times, two layers of metaphor were added to the term: the first referred to bodily signs of holy grace . . . [stigmata]; the second, a medical allusion to this religious allusion, referred to bodily signs of physical disorder. Today, the term is widely used in something like the original literal sense, but is applied more to the disgrace itself than to the bodily evidence of it [Goffman, 1963: 1–2].

Visibility of the evidence, however, remains the foundation on which stigma is built. To be disgraced there must be some available grounds.

When evidence takes the form of physical signs of disorder, weakness, or moral or physical pathology, questions about how the disgrace is discovered are moot. Attention turns to the consequences of this public evidence for the stigmatized and for others—to how people cope with disgrace. Goffman calls these the concerns of the *discredited*. For instance, we saw in Chapter Six how people attempted to mend and restore face or reputation in the wake of a public seizure.

Goffman details a distinct and equally insightful set of concerns that face those for whom the evidence of a putatively devaluing quality is not so visible. This is the situation of the *discreditable*, those for whom the primary problem is controlling information about these aspects of self. When this information can be kept secret, others are likely to warrant what Goffman calls one's "virtual" self, namely, the normal, regular person we present ourselves to be among other normal, regular persons. In an interactional sense, such persons *are* normals, which is to say free of disgrace and stigma. The concept of stigma in sociological writing has been extended to include the discreditable with the discredited.

The situation of people with epilepsy is routinely that of the discreditable, punctuated periodically for most by specifically discrediting public seizures. But seizures are not directly analogous to the cuts, burns, stigmata, or physical handicaps and disfigurements Goffman discusses. While many people believe their seizures to be "blemishes of individual character" in others' eyes, seizures are in fact not a form of evidence that is always or even routinely available to others. Some people almost never have seizures; others only during their sleep or upon waking; others only rarely, and in forms that are easily normalized or neutralized. Even those who have many grand mal seizures are otherwise perfectly normal in appearance (perhaps a bit less so in terms of social participation). Because such evidence is stigmatizing and yet frequently manipulatable, controlling knowledge of one's epilepsy becomes as important as controlling seizures themselves.

We use the term "stigma potential" to highlight the contingent nature of this feared disgrace by epilepsy. Describing the stigma as potential assumes that knowledge of one's epilepsy is limited to few others, and that if it were to become more widely known, significant redefinition of self, accompanied by various restrictions on and regulation of conduct, might follow. This assumption was held rather widely, in varying degree, among the people we interviewed. Goffman suggests that such discreditable attributes weigh heavily and shamefully on one's own definitions of self, quite aside from others knowing. We prefer to leave that question open, to be determined through studying specific cases. Howard Becker (1963, 1973) has discussed what he calls the "secret" or "potential" deviant as one who (1) recognizes his or her own acts, qualities, and characteristics *and* (2) is aware of certain relevant prohibitions extant in the larger cultural and social setting. Given this knowledge, he or she concludes that there is at least some probability—varying by the particulars of the situation—that disclosure would lead to discrediting and undesirable consequences. Becker is more equivocal than Goffman on the issue of self derogation and shame, requiring only that the individual be aware that rules do exist that may be applied and enforced by others, were they to learn of the hidden practice or attribute. Although shame is an important phenomenon, it is not a necessary precondition to the rise of information control strategies. Even those who decried public stereotypes of and discrimination toward people with epilepsy were sensitive to the practical wisdom of keeping their epilepsy secret in some situations.

THE PERCEPTION OF STIGMA *

Stigma, then, is by no means an automatic result of possessing some discreditable attribute. The impact and meaning of stigma linked to epilepsy in one's life is the product of a definitional process involving the individual

---

*The balance of this chapter contains expanded and altered segments from Schneider and Conrad (1980).

and various others across a range of social situations and settings. While we may speak of disrepute attached to some general quality or characteristic, we must look to the details of the specific case before concluding that stigma is experienced and how this happens (cf. P. West, 1982; Ryan et al., 1980). What the individual thinks about him or herself, as well as about what others think, is crucial. A discreditable attribute or performance becomes relevant to self only if the individual perceives it as discreditable, whether or not such perceptions actually exist among others. In short, the individual has an important hand in constructing the stigma of epilepsy and the moral meanings surrounding illness more generally. It is even possible that people considered "ill" by others are themselves unaware of such attributions of meaning: for instance the person perplexed by sympathetic reactions to his or her disclosure of cancer, or the young "tough" who in polite society wears venereal disease as a badge of sexual prowess.

Most sociological work on stigma assumes that the stigmatized learn the negative meaning of their attribute or performance primarily through direct exposure to rejection and disapproval from others. There is, however, little research that examines actual *interactions* between such people and "normals." Similarly poorly understood is the *perception* of stigma (see P. West, 1982), of what the putatively stigmatized think others think of them and "their kind," and how these others *might* react to disclosure. This brings us back to the situation of Goffman's discreditable person, but makes the individual's own definitions of self and others central and problematic. We believe it is from these definitions of others' definitions and actions that stigma is constructed.

Two pervasive themes in our respondents' comments are that they "have" something that others "don't understand," and that this lack of understanding and knowledge of "what epilepsy is" is a fundamental source of others' negative reactions. The little information others have about epilepsy is thought probably to be incorrect and stereotypical, sometimes incorporating elements of madness and evil. As we have shown, our respondents described others' reactions to epilepsy with the adjectives "frightened" and "scared." One woman, diagnosed at middle age and who had lost a teaching job because of seizures at work, said:

> Well, I understand it now and *I'm* not afraid of it. But most people are unless they've experienced it, and so you just don't talk to other people about it, and if you do, never use the word "epilepsy." The word itself, I mean job-ways, insurance-ways . . . anything, the hang-ups there are on it. There's just too much prejudice so the less said about it the better.

One man compared others' ignorance and fear of epilepsy to similar reactions to leprosy: "The public is so illy-educated toward an epileptic. It's like someone with leprosy walking into a room. You see a leper and you run because you're afraid of it." A woman spoke of the "historical implications" of epilepsy:

> The fact of *having* epilepsy. It isn't the seizures. I think they are a very minor part of it. Its implication[s] are so *enormous*. The historical implications of epilepsy are fantastic. I'm lucky to have been born when I was. If I was born at the beginning of this century I would have been discarded . . . probably locked away somewhere.

People with epilepsy see its public image tainted by ignorance and fear. These perceptions become grist for decisions and strategies about the importance of keeping such discrediting information secret.

Not surprisingly, the possibility of public seizures was a source of great concern for those who believed epilepsy to be disreputable. One woman said seizures are "like having your pants fall down" in public. Another young woman described others' view of seizures: "I can't use the word 'horrible,' but they think . . . it's *ugly*. It is. It's strange. It's

something you're not used to seeing." The visual events
that make up seizures, including loss of consciousness, violent muscle contractions, falling to the ground, or simply
being "absent" from the social scene, become the objec-
tive evidence for a more fundamental, "essential" disreputability. Another woman said:

It's one of those fear images; it's something that people don't know about and it has strong negative con-
notations in people's minds. It's a bad image, something scary, sort of like a beggar; it's dirty, the person
falling down and frothing at the mouth and jerking
and the bystanders not knowing what to do. It's something that happens in public which isn't nice.

Whether or not these people label themselves negatively,
or feel shame, they perceive the social meanings of epilepsy and seizures as threats to their status as normal, competent, and equal members of society. To the extent they
held such views of others' definitions of epilepsy, they took
pains to conceal their condition in these situations.

STRATEGIES OF SELECTIVE
CONCEALMENT

Given the view of the social landscape our respondents
held, we might expect them to conceal their epilepsy
across virtually all of their relationships and throughout
the course of their lives. But their strategies of managing
information were rarely so simple. Sometimes people concealed their epilepsy, sometimes they did not, and the
same persons could be both open and closed about it at a
single period in their lives. Moreover, concealment and
disclosure often were matters of degree that varied over
time and particular experience. In short, people managed
information about epilepsy in ways contingent on situation, others involved, and potential consequences of concealment or disclosure.

A part of the wisdom of the world of epilepsy is that

there are some people you can tell and others you cannot. Even among the most secretive (six of our respondents said we were the first people they had told or talked with about epilepsy outside their physicians and immediate families; one woman said that her parents, her physician, and we were the only people who knew of her epilepsy, and that she had kept it secret even from her husband of seventeen years), at least a handful of others know of their condition. Close friends and family members are most often in this category of safe others who can be told, supplemented by people one can "feel comfortable with," and those who "won't react negatively to epilepsy."

These safe family members and friends often were used to "test the waters" of reaction: "I think the first couple of times I mentioned it was with my very closest friends to sort of test the water. When it wasn't any problem, then I began to feel freer to mention it." Wider disclosure depended on how these early tests went. If people began to sense negative consequences from such telling, typically they returned to concealment as the predominant way to control the impact of epilepsy in their lives. One woman said, for example:

> I tried to get a driver's license when I was eighteen or nineteen, after I was married. We were living in Mississippi and I put it on [the form] that I was epileptic, only because I was afraid if I pass out and I'm drivin' a car, well, that's dangerous. I took the thing up there and they said, "Epileptics can't—you have to have a doctor's thing." We moved about two months later to California. I got my driver's license and didn't put it down.

She made some initial attempts at disclosure, including a college dormitory application that resulted in this woman being disqualified from living on campus and, in consequence, declining a scholarship. She concluded that secrecy was the only strategy to minimize the risk of rejection and discriminatory treatment. She said, recalling these events: "I don't know if maybe I wasn't testing . . . at the time, you know, well, 'Is it okay?' If things had been different, maybe I could have talked about it." We asked another woman if she discusses epilepsy with new people she meets. She said:

> It depends. I still find it hard, but I'm trying to. I have to trust somebody a lot before I'll tell them in terms of a friendship basis. All my close friends know, but in terms of my work, forget it. This is a risk I can't take after the [previous] experience. I still have great inbuilt fears about losing a job from it. I'm not ready to put myself at that risk.

And an upwardly mobile young administrator said he lost his driver's license as a result of disclosing his epilepsy. He recalled that experience and what he had learned from it: "I started out tryin' to be honest about it and got burned. So I gave up bein' honest about it in that circumstance." Although this man did disclose his epilepsy to a wide variety of others, including his employer, he said he regularly lied about it on driver's license forms.

People can and do maintain carefully segregated and selective strategies of managing the stigma potential of epilepsy. Some situations were considered of higher risk than others. Concealing epilepsy in employment interviews, including directly lying about it, even after they were hired, was spoken of often. Some feared reprisal if their employer later discovered their epilepsy. They recommended a strategy of monitoring the interview to "see how it's going." If they saw approval in others' reactions to them, once initial contact was made, they said they might try disclosure. One young woman who said she had not had a seizure for nineteen years and took no medication was still very sensitive about her "past" when it came to applying for a job:

> Well, employers are the only thing I haven't been open with. On an application, I will not write it. If I feel I have a chance for a job and I'm gonna make it, I'll bring it up. But to put it on that application—be-

cause employers, they look at it, they see that thing checked; it just gives me a feeling that they don't give you a chance.

Although she had never experienced discriminatory treatment in employment, this woman usually waits, she said, "until I get into that interview and sell myself first. Then I'll come out and say, 'There's one more point . . .'" Another respondent said he would wait until "I have my foot in the door and they said, 'Hey, he's doing okay'" before disclosing his epilepsy to employers. This strategy of gradual disclosure in the face of growing rapport with employers sometimes led to surprised reactions that others made so little of their condition. As a result of such experience, our respondents proceeded to redefine, at least in part, their ideas of others' reactions to epilepsy as well as their own ways of coping.

Finally, it was important to conceal epilepsy in situations where others might be predisposed to criticize. A woman who was open with friends said she would not want others in her neighborhood to know. She explained: "At this point I'm not involved in quarrels. I would think that if I got into a quarrel or feuding situation, it [the epilepsy] would be something that would be used against me." This view of epilepsy as ammunition in critics' hands was reiterated by a man who defined his work as "very political." He said if his critics learned of his epilepsy, they would "add that on as an element of [my] character that makes [me] undesirable." Sometimes concealment against adversaries can exclude those who otherwise would be told. One woman said because her brother had married a woman she did not particularly like, she had decided simply not to tell him of her diagnosis. She said of her sister-in-law, "She's the type that would [say,] you know, 'you're crazy because you have it,' or 'there's something wrong with you.' And she would probably laugh." Finally, even one's physician may be defined more as an official gatekeeper than an advocate and counselor. One man said:

If he is going to go running to the state and tell the
state every time I have a seizure, I don't feel I can be
honest with that doctor. He is not keeping his part of
the bargain. Everything on my medical records are
supposed to be sacred.

These stories demonstrate how the idea of being open
or closed about some putatively stigmatizing quality blurs
much rich detail in how people actually manage such information. Moreover, being open or closed about epilepsy
or, for that matter, other potentially discrediting attributes,
can have little to do with one's identity. Those who conceal may do so on wholly practical grounds, based on their
own past experience or beliefs. Such disclosure and concealment appear contingent upon a complex interaction of
one's learned perceptions of the stigma of epilepsy, actual
experiences with others that follow disclosure, and the nature of the particular relationships involved.

INSTRUMENTAL TELLING: DISCLOSING AS A MANAGEMENT STRATEGY

Managing information, even when the information is
potentially discrediting, can include disclosure as well as
concealment. With the exception of perhaps nine or ten
respondents who adopted the most rigidly secretive strategies, our respondents said they "usually" or "always" told
certain others of their epilepsy under *certain* circumstances. Disclosure was virtually always described as serv-
ing some end. Two goals were mentioned most often:
telling as "therapy," and telling to prevent various consequences believed worse than the possible stigma of disclosure. Like the strategies of concealment we discussed
earlier, this kind of telling attempts to mitigate the potentially negative impact of epilepsy and others' definitions of
it on one's self and daily round. In short, this telling is
instrumental.

Disclosing feelings of guilt, culpability, and self-derogation can be cathartic, as we know from much social science research. Such telling can serve a therapeutic function for the individual by sharing or diffusing the burden of these feelings, particularly for those who have concealed what they see as some personal blemish or flaw. It can free the energy used to control information for other social activities. This therapy, however, depends on the availability of the properly receptive audience, i.e., those willing to be supportive, encouraging, empathetic, and/or nonjudgmental. Beyond catharsis, such occasions of telling become grounds for people to develop definitions of their condition as an unremarkable and neutral (perhaps even "interesting," as one man said) facet of themselves. This sort of telling as therapy is akin to what Fred Davis (1961) described as the relief associated with "breaking through" the silence surrounding interactions of physically disabled polio victims and so-called normals.

Therapeutic telling is instrumental, then, primarily in its salutary impact on the actor's self definition, or at minimum, in simply sharing important information about self. Those who recalled telling select and safe others said that just being able to talk about epilepsy was important. One woman said of such talking, "It's what's got me together about it [the epilepsy]." A man recalled how telling friends about epilepsy allowed him to minimize it in his own mind:

I think in talking to them [friends] I would try to convince myself that it didn't have to be terribly important. Now that I think more about it, I was probably just defiant about it: "I ain't gonna let this God-damned thing get in my way, period."

And finally, one of the few respondents who had told virtually no one, in keeping with her mother's careful coaching, suggested how she might use our interview as grounds for redefining her epilepsy and self:

It just seems so weird now that I've—because I'm talking to you about it, and I've never talked to anybody about it. It's really not so bad. You know it hasn't affected me that much, but no one wants to talk about it. . . . [Talking about epilepsy] makes me feel I'm really not so bad off. Just because I can't find answers to those questions, cuz like I think I feel sorry for myself. I can sit around the house and just dream up all these things, you know, why I'm so persecuted and [all].

Selective disclosure to supportive and nonjudgmental others can thus help "banish the ghosts" that flourish in secrecy and isolation. It allows for feedback and the renegotiation of the perception of stigma. Through externalizing what is believed to be a potentially negative feature of self, people with epilepsy and their audiences redefine this attribute as an "ordinary" part of themselves. We saw this same settling, comforting reaction earlier, in the "relief" of knowing one's diagnosis. Thus, for many people, knowing and then disclosing one's epilepsy were crucial steps toward greater independence from the social and personal implications of the condition. This strategy appears effective, however, primarily among one's intimates and close friends. Particularly when facing strangers or those whose reactions cannot be assumed supportive, such as prospective employers, the motor vehicle bureau, or virtually any bureaucracy's application form, this openness can be set aside quickly in preference for a thoroughgoing secrecy.

A second kind of instrumental telling we call "preventive": disclosure to influence others' actions and/or ideas toward the individual and toward those with epilepsy in general. Respondents sometimes said they disclosed their epilepsy to those with whom they shared some routine, and who, as a result, might more likely witness one of their seizures. The grounds cited for this telling are that others then "will know what it is" and "won't be scared."

This anticipatory preventive telling offers a kind of "medical disclaimer" (cf. Hewitt and Stokes, 1975). By bringing a blameless, beyond-my-control medical frame to such potentially discrediting events, people attempt to reduce the risk that more morally disreputable interpretations might be applied by naïve witnesses. One young woman recalled that she felt "great" when her parents told her junior high teachers about epilepsy. She said, "I'd rather have them know than think I was a dummy or something . . . or think I was having . . . you know, *problems*." Reflecting the power of medical excuse (as well as a relative hierarchy of legitimacy among medical excuses), a middle-aged man who described himself as an "alcoholic" told of how he would disclose epilepsy to defuse others' complaints about his drinking:

> I'd say, "I have to drink. It's the only way I can maintain . . . I have seizures you know" . . . and this kind of thing. People would then feel embarrassed. Or you'd say, "I'm epileptic," then they'd feel embarrassed and say, "Oh, well, gee, we're sorry, that's right. We forgot about that."

This account and similar ones illustrate the kind of social currency medical definitions possess, both for illness in general and for epilepsy in particular. As with all currency, however, its effectiveness as a medium of acceptable exchange rests on whether others will accept it as worthy. What others in fact think of such medical accounts remains, unfortunately, unknown.

Beyond providing a medical frame through which others will interpret seizures, preventive telling may include specific instructions about what to do in case of a seizure. Since our respondents believed others to be almost totally ignorant of what seizures are, they assumed them to have little idea of how to react. By providing what are, in effect, directions, respondents tried to protect both their bodies and their selves. The young public administrator we quoted earlier said:

> Down the road, I'll usually make a point to tell someone I'm around a lot because I know that it's frighten-

ing, so I will partly for my own purposes, tell them
I've got it—if I have one [seizure] that it's nothing to
worry about. And don't take me to the hospital even if
I ask you to. I always tell people that I work with because I presume I'll be with them for some long period of time. And I may have a seizure and I want
them to know what not to do in particular.

People believed such telling solved some problems for
naïve others. While these others have the responsibility of
carrying out the instructions—which, recall, are typically
"do nothing," "don't call the ambulance," and "keep me
from hurting myself"—such directions would seem to
shift the authority and therefore the moral responsibility
back to the person with epilepsy. Whether or not witnesses would agree we simply cannot say.

People also may disclose their epilepsy to those who
appear to be candidates for close relationships in order to
minimize the pain of later rejection. As one man said, "If
they're going to leave [because of epilepsy], better it be
sooner than later." Another spoke of such telling as a "good
way of testing" what kind of friend such persons would be.
He said, "Why go through all the trauma of falling in love
with someone if they are going to hate your guts once they
find out you're an epileptic?"

Moreover, we discovered that people disclose their epilepsy to "educate" others. While this strategy is sometimes mediated by and supported through participation in
various self-help groups, it also is initiated directly by individuals. One young man who became active in a local self-
help group described his "rap" on epilepsy as follows:

It's a good manner. I use it quite a bit. I'll come
through and say epilepsy is a condition, not a disease.
I can throw out all the statistics. I usually say most
people are not in wheelchairs or in bed because of
epilepsy, they're walking the streets just like I am and
other people. Anything like that to make comparisons,
to get a point across.

Another respondent, who said she had herself benefited greatly by an early talk with a veteran epileptic, spoke of the importance of such education: "That's why I think it is important to come out of the closet to some extent. Because once people have met an epileptic and found out that it's a *person* with epilepsy, that helps a lot." As this woman suggests, perhaps independent of the *content* of the disclosure, exposure to a person who, among other things, "has epilepsy" may become grist for others' redefinition not only of that person but of "epileptics" more generally.

In sum, for those who possess some discreditable feature of self, some generally hidden "fact" or quality, the disclosure of which they believe will bring undesired consequences, a major strategy is to attempt to control information. In this chapter we have described how people with epilepsy manage this. Our analysis uncovers some of the complexity of how people parcel out or withhold discrediting information about themselves. In addition, we have noted how telling or disclosing can serve the same ends as concealing.

EIGHT

Ties That Bind and Free: The Paradox of Medical Care

Doctors help people who have an illness maintain conventional lives. People with epilepsy rely on doctors to make proper diagnoses, provide information, give support and direction in managing epilepsy, and to prescribe and monitor medications that help control seizures. They *need* physicians to help them control epilepsy. At the same time, our respondents had distinctly mixed feelings about their relationships with doctors. Some respondents characterized their doctors as "conscientious," "gentle and caring," "supportive," and said they were "satisfied" and "treated well." Others complained about doctors who "didn't care," or who were "brusque," "always in a hurry," and "very little help." Some said they were "frustrated" with their medical care and had "very little relationship" with their physicians. In this chapter we explore some sources of this ambivalence and describe the experience our respondents had with doctors and medicine.

SEEKING INFORMATION

Patients look to doctors not only for treatment but for correct information about epilepsy and its impact on their future. Our respondents spoke often about how limited and vague the information was that their doctors provided. Those who expressed this view were more likely also to feel unsupported and personally dissatisfied with medical care than those who saw doctor-provided information as adequate and complete.

Information in the doctor-patient relationship must flow in both directions: it is of value to both parties. Patients give the doctors information about their life and body troubles. Doctors evaluate and process this (as well as other) information to make a diagnosis and plan treatment; they then return medically-informed judgment to patients in the form of advice, treatment regimens, and prognosis. Information is a currency on which this relationship depends. But our respondents said they often felt they gave more information than they received. Sociological studies document that doctors limit or control the amount of information shared with patients. It is information about prognosis that seems to be shared with patients most selectively (Glaser and Strauss, 1965; Davis, 1963; Roth, 1963), especially with the chronically ill. Control of information, however, is practiced in many if not most encounters between patients and doctors (Quint, 1965; Danziger, 1978). Physicians seem to give relatively little time to providing medical information and answering questions, at least to their patients' satisfaction (C. West,

1982). One study reported that one minute of a twenty minute appointment was given to transmitting information to patients (Waitzkin, 1976).

Sociologists have offered various explanations for such information control by physicians. One suggested source is what Talcott Parsons (1951) called the asymmetric or unbalanced relationship between doctor and patient. The medical profession has a socially warranted monopoly on medical knowledge and expertise (Freidson, 1970). Doctors are the authorities in the world of medicine. This produces a situation defined primarily by doctors' questions and patients' responses. Sandra Danziger (1978) and Candace West (1983) studied how physicians manage information to maintain control of patient-physician encounters. Others (e.g., Waitzkin, 1976) argue that control of information is what reproduces the institutional power of the doctor over the patient.

The control of information has more immediate functions than reflecting and maintaining these differences in power and status (see also Skipper et al., 1964). One sociologist suggests that physicians limit information about prognosis because they are unsure of the patient's emotional reaction or of the patient's ability to understand the information, because they do not want to remove hope, or because they want the patient to make the best of a situation (Davis, 1963). Discussing certain problems may make health professionals themselves anxious, so they withhold information and avoid specific discussions (Quint, 1965). Many doctors have very busy practices and see information sharing as a secondary task to first-rate medical treatment. There is some evidence that doctors may underestimate patients' abilities to comprehend medical information (McKinlay, 1972) and, as a result, offer very little. Current medical education gives little emphasis to giving patients information as compared to, say, taking a history. Very little attention is paid to preparing doctors to handle the social and emotional aspects of medical care (Coombs, 1978).

These and similar factors may contribute to the unhappiness with the amount and depth of information provided by doctors and other medical personnel.

INFORMATION: A SCARCE
AND VALUABLE RESOURCE

To people with epilepsy, information about it is a vital resource in managing their lives. A diagnosis gives problems or unexplained experiences a handle, but alone says little about what epilepsy is, what might happen, and what should be done. Information about the disorder can help locate the person's experience in the medical and social world. It can alleviate fears, dispel misconceptions, and give people greater understanding of their troubles. By understanding the vicissitudes of epilepsy, sufferers can better comprehend what is happening to them and perhaps feel more in control of their lives.

To the extent that doctors offered our respondents specific information, they appear to have done so in early encounters. After the initial diagnosis and first few appointments, visits to the doctor become routine. Doctors ask questions such as "How are you doing—any seizures?," give a brief physical examination, and prescribe a refill of medication. Unless a patient presents a specific problem or change in condition (an increase in seizures, bad headaches, new medication side effects, etc.), the doctor-patient encounter is brief, routine, and not an occasion for conveying new information to the patient. Doctors rarely ask patients if *they* have any questions or inquire about the effects of epilepsy on their everyday lives. Doctors at a university medical center and a county hospital were perceived as very busy and always in a hurry. Patients are reluctant to infringe on their time with "personal" questions. The doctor-patient encounter becomes largely a technical check up, focusing on the body as machine and bypassing the person with the disorder. Patients can interrupt this

routine, but only with difficulty. One articulate professional woman shared her predicament:

> It's just very professional and businesslike. They often
> take another EEG to see what's going on and ask me,
> "Well, when was the last time you had a convulsion
> and are you having any problems with your medica-
> tion? Do you feel like you're overmedicated? Can you
> still concentrate and function normally? Oh, fine. See
> you in six months." And so it's been real hard for me
> to be assertive and say, "Well, I need more than that.
> You know, can I ask you some questions?" And I did
> get to the point where I would write down questions
> and take them with me cuz I'd just get so flustered. I
> really get intimidated by them you know, walking in,
> walking out. . . . That did help.

The information doctors were reported to have given
our respondents ranged widely in amount and substance.
Some said they obtained none at all, most believed they received too little, and a few reported they got full descriptions of the disorder. Information varied according to such
factors as the doctor's professional stance, the patient's age,
the type of epilepsy, and the patient's facility in asking the
doctor questions. Correlations between information received and these "variables" need not concern us here,
beyond noting that information exchange and reception
were not completely uniform. What is of greater importance is that there appears to be a clear and definite skew-
ing toward the "little information" end of the spectrum
and that very few patients believed they got as much information as they wanted.

Children experience particular blocks to information.
Medical convention suggests that parents ought to be talked
to privately by doctors about their child's problem. It may
be that doctors believe children incapable of understanding what is said, or that children should be protected from
knowing the details of their disorder, or that parents are
the most appropriate conveyors of information to minors.

Reasons aside, doctors usually bypass children when discussing their disorders. This effectively limits the child's access to information. As we discussed in Chapter Three, children receive most of their information from a parent.

Young children are not alone in being denied access to information. One woman diagnosed at thirteen said no one even mentioned the word epilepsy to her until she was sixteen. One young man's doctor would not see him without his parents until he was twenty-one years old. He said the information he received was very limited: "[The doctor] never related any real information. He was [a] . . . very conservative gentleman. And when I turned eighteen, he said, 'You have to listen to the four Ds: no drinking, no driving, no drugs, and no draft.'" Teenagers resent being treated as if they were still children who need to be protected. Adolescence is a time of expanding personal independence. One young man told us, "The first neurologist I did not like because I don't think he treated me like a person. It was more like a little kid coming in. I was thirteen and able to understand and felt I had a right to know 'cuz I was the one who had it."

Beyond "just take your pills," many children were told that there was a possibility they might outgrow epilepsy. Either through the adults' manipulation of information or through their own selective memories, some children receive a distorted impression of this possibility. One woman said that when she was a child, her doctor told her she "might outgrow it [or] . . . might not. It might get worse. The medicine could probably control it . . . mostly pretty hopeful [stuff]."

Such a possibility, while hopeful, can create a whole new set of uncertainties (see Comaroff and Maguire, 1981). How old must one be to outgrow it? If one does not have seizures does this mean the medication is working or that one has outgrown the problem? A subsequent seizure creates a letdown and disappointment, along with the hope that this one will be the last. The person must ask, How long will this continue? After being told she had epilepsy, one woman asked her doctor:

"Well, how long am I going to have it?" and he said, "For about a year." . . . He told me [that at] the mild stage it was, some people outgrow it within a year. . . . I haven't. [He also said] there may be a chance I could be on these pills for the rest of my life.

Only two or three of our respondents could have outgrown their epilepsy (although some people, especially those diagnosed as children, do).* Many said it took years before they stopped expecting each year to be the year they would outgrow it.

There also was a clear sense among those diagnosed as adults that the quality and quantity of information received was deficient. One 40-year-old man recalled an early encounter that was to typify subsequent experience with his doctor:

You'd sit down and talk with him and he'd take notes and ask you how you were feeling and I guess he was trying to explain to me what it was, but he never did explain what it was. He explained how to live with it and asked how are you living with it? But I didn't know—I know how I was living, but I didn't know what I was living with because no one ever explained that. To this day I couldn't tell you what type of epilepsy I have.

Although this doctor *did* provide information about epilepsy, it did not, at least in this man's eyes, answer the most important question: "What *is* epilepsy?"

Some patients did ask doctors questions about the origins and consequences of epilepsy. Many also sought information elsewhere, especially in books. One young man's doctor never talked to him about epilepsy until he started asking questions at fourteen: "I just kept waiting for some-

---

*This small number may be due to our sampling strategy. People who outgrew epilepsy may not present themselves to researchers soliciting "people with epilepsy."

body to tell me about it and they never would, so I figured I'd better ask." But with little understanding of epilepsy to begin with, it is difficult to formulate the most pertinent questions. As a part-time college instructor said, "I didn't know enough even to know what questions to ask. You can't ask a doctor, 'Well, if A, should I B?' unless you know B exists." Information then becomes the wellspring for seeking more information.

Of course, not all physicians withhold information about epilepsy from their patients. Many doctors give out different amounts or kinds of information in different ways and in different circumstances. Typically, doctors explain briefly what the disorder is and that it usually *can* be controlled medically. They might also give prescriptive information about what one should do: take medications, sit or lie down if one feels a seizure coming, call the doctor if one has an abnormal number of seizures, go for check ups regularly, watch for side effects of medications, and so forth. Sometimes patients are told to avoid certain situations, such as getting overtired or overstressed, drinking to excess, rooms with strobe lights, and the like. Doctors may mention possible restrictions on driving, swimming, and certain kinds of work. Occasionally, a person recalled that a doctor explained the results of an EEG examination.

Our respondents appreciated doctors who were straightforward in presenting information. A 19-year-old factory worker remarked, "He was a pretty good doctor. He sort of tried to explain it to me. Told me to stay calm about it, what it was like." When we asked about his current doctor, he said, "Oh, he's a pretty square shooter, you know, something you don't understand, you can go up and talk to him." A 35-year-old welfare worker appreciated his doctors' attempt to outline the potential problems he might face: "Basically they've been honest about it. They've told me what the story is and tried to explain what possible limitations I might have."

Information comes in a variety of packages. As patients

see it, some physicians give out specific recipes of information depicting what patients should do, such as the "4 Ds" mentioned above, or "healthy habits" that should be followed. One woman said her doctor "explained that I did need to have my sleep, to eat a good balanced diet, not to skip meals 'cuz that has a tendency to throw you." Another middle-aged woman felt supported when her doctor minimized the possible consequences of epilepsy. Her neurologist joked with her, telling her lots of people, including Caesar and Van Gogh had epilepsy and that she "shouldn't worry about it too much." She thought his attitude was "great."

But even respondents who told us their doctors provided them much information, often suggested that this had not always been the case. Frequently, these respondents had had earlier less satisfying medical experiences. A young woman said, "I think in fact that he sat down with me and was the first doctor that ever sat down and explained to me as an adult and made me understand." A 19-year-old man recalled:

My doctor in [home city] that treated me first didn't tell me much at all. The one in [big city] I went to . . . probably explained more to me. He really laid it on the line. He told me it was like a . . . disorder of the nervous system and . . . there were a lot of people who have it. . . . And he said, "You can just live a normal life, the only thing is to keep on medication."

Among these patients the information exchange was more balanced (although most still said they received less than they would have liked). This exchange represented a give and take, with patients and doctors both asking and responding in turn.

In a very few instances (four out of eighty), patients and doctors engaged in a type of mutual participation (cf. Szsaz and Hollender, 1956) as coparticipants in treatment (cf. Danziger, 1978). In addition to reducing the dependency inherent in the doctor-patient relationship, this cooperation encourages consideration of the social context of seizure occurrences. Doctors may see this cooperation as more appropriate for specific forms of epilepsy—three of our four coparticipating respondents had psychomotor or "psychological" seizures.

One woman and her doctor together concluded that some of her seizures were "psychological":

So [the doctor] and I talked. And then I did a lot of research on epilepsy on my own. Not to sit down and memorize all, but enough to educate myself. And I have come to the conclusion that some of my seizures are psychological, but there are still some that aren't. The usual way I can tell . . . whether they are psychological or not is whether I have an aura ahead of time.

A young professional man with psychomotor seizures described his most recent doctor's appointment:

I just saw him today at 1:30. At first we go through . . . medication and then we go through things which are happening like how many episodes I've had and what happens before and after and how I feel and what kind of activities I've done before and trying to correlate them to find out where the episodes come from . . . which is very fundamental in psychomotor epilepsy, to find out where they came from.

Doctors who take such a coparticipant stance make the patient an active partner in treatment, rather than merely expecting the patient to take medications and come regularly for check ups. These patients, although few in number, were among the most positive about their relationships with their doctor and "most satisfied" with the quantity and quality of information received. It seems the more a patient knows about epilepsy, the better he or she is able to manage the disorder; the more information that is doctor-rendered the more positive the experience of the doctor-patient relationship.*

* There are exceptions, of course. One woman has not talked to her doctor about epilepsy for sixteen or seventeen years. "I see a doctor to

One final point. We have been talking about doctors as though they are perceived to be the same but they are not. Such analysis masks significant variation. People with epilepsy may see both neurologists and family doctors for medical care of their disorder. Family doctors are perceived to be more concerned, supportive, and forthcoming with information than neurologists, especially about life issues involved in managing epilepsy. But family doctors actually know relatively little about the intricacies of the medico-technological aspects of epilepsy—diagnostic differentiations, types of seizures, and varieties and dosages of medications. Many people themselves came to this conclusion and were referred to or went to see neurologists. When patients visit specialists, however, the balance of the already asymmetric doctor-patient relationship tips even further. People sometimes expect specialists to minister to all their medical care needs, but the province of the specialist, at least in this case, remains disproportionately medico-technological. Neurologists treat the seizure disorder, but not the person with epilepsy. There is a certain irony here. Family doctors are seen to give information but they have little; neurologists have information but they give little. Where do patients turn?

OBTAINING INFORMATION

Patients' general dissatisfaction with the amount and kind of information shared affects how they view their doctor. Patients may conclude that physicians neither know nor want to know much about epilepsy. One woman who "never talked to any doctor much about epilepsy" concluded, "I think doctors are rather uninformed, just like the rest of us are. . . . Or if they were informed, they didn't let me know." Patients also may conclude that doctors are

---

get my prescription refilled. . . . I've never asked him about epilepsy; I don't want to talk about it."

aloof and distant, or that they do not really care about the patient's problems. While they remain dependent on doctors for medical care and medications, their negative impressions increase their ambivalence toward medicine.

When they feel the medical world has failed them, patients give up on doctors as a source of information and look elsewhere (see Stewart and Sullivan, 1982; Comaroff and Maguire, 1981). People with epilepsy turn to libraries, magazines, medical books, the national epilepsy society, and, occasionally, to other epileptics. Two stories are exemplary. The first, from a man:

[After not getting much information from my doctor] I went out and tried to find out on my own what it was. Then I was a psychiatric technician at [the hospital] . . . for a little over a year. I used to take people down to get EEGs and it's kind of interesting because I looked in these books, volumes on different types of epilepsy, and I didn't realize how many different kinds of epilepsy there were. And I kept looking for my kind.

A woman said, "[My doctor] just told me what it was like . . . a short circuit in your electrical circuit . . . that everything just went haywire and that's why it happened."

We asked if her doctor gave her any information about managing epilepsy. She said:

No, he just told me to take my medication and that's about it. I was talking to my mom about it and she said that the only way we were really going to find out about epilepsy is to write one of the leagues of epilepsy . . . and they sent out pamphlets and stuff. I was calling hospitals and everything and they couldn't tell me anything.

Given this dissatisfaction, it is reasonable to ask what it is these patients want from their doctors. What kind of information do they want? Beyond a medical handle for their problem (a diagnosis) and professional aid in controlling their seizures (prescribed medications), patients want explanations of what epilepsy is, what is happening to them, what might happen, and how they might better manage epilepsy and its impact on their lives. They want to be listened to, supported through their fears, and helped to make better adaptations. They want doctors to *share* more with them. For some this is very general: "If someone had just sat down and said *anything* [about epilepsy and what was happening] to me, I would have been so grateful at that point." For others it can be very specific, as one woman explained:

My GP tries to be supportive, he's just real rushed. He gives hugs and stuff and that's like a real daddy kind of person. But they don't really sit down and look at you . . . and say, "Hey, you're an intelligent person and you wanna know what's going on in your head with that seizure. What it is and what it's not." They try to allay your fears without real explanations. I wanted them to tell me [the] kinds of things I've seen in the literature. What a seizure is and basically, more important, what a seizure is not. I think that's the biggest fear I have. Can I die? Can I choke? Can I . . . ? Oh, big fears. I wanted my bigger fears allayed without [him] then saying, "Well, go for another blood test."

Knowledge and understanding are resources that enable people to deal better with having epilepsy. They may contribute to new management strategies that foster greater independence. A woman said:

I wish they would have told me more, explained to me what epilepsy was because maybe then it could have helped a little more because once I explained the situation, or they explained the situation to me, and explained to me the differences in seizures . . . I felt I was much more equipped to handle them.

Our respondents wanted their doctors to be allies in the struggle to control the impact of epilepsy (and not seizures alone) in their lives. For whatever reasons, doctors were seen this way only occasionally by the people we interviewed.

GAINING CONTROL

Gaining control over epilepsy is a many-layered process. First comes discovering what is happening to one's body. Once that is established (as a diagnosis), control of seizures and contending with the new status as "epileptic" become predominant. But for many, seizure control is imperfect. They may continue having seizures albeit at a greatly reduced rate. Both medications and life regimens are believed critical to controlling seizures. Moreover, gaining control over epilepsy involves more than controlling seizures. One must have knowledge about how to manage the social experience of epilepsy.

Knowledge then is a resource for developing ways to manage one's life. It includes acknowledging and validating one's feelings about epilepsy, learning how to minimize the interference of seizures and stigma in one's life, managing medications and other regimens, and dealing with other people and their reactions. Finally, people gain control of epilepsy by controlling information, both by concealing it and sharing it (see Chapter Seven). Patients, at least initially, are almost as dependent on doctors for this information as they are for their medication prescriptions.

The work of gaining control of epilepsy is an ongoing struggle. Our respondents' ambivalence toward medical care stemmed from a perception that their doctors had in part failed them. They believed their doctors had little comprehension of their struggle and of how to be an ally. Doctors' concerns with diagnosis and seizure control are appreciated, but the patient's struggle with epilepsy extends well beyond the clinic. Here doctors are of little help. The struggle belongs to the patient. In one sense that is as it should be. Like everyone else, people with epilepsy are ultimately responsible for managing their own lives. But managing epilepsy as a disorder is too narrowly defined as a medical task, and most doctors see their medical treatment as ending with diagnosis, medications, and routine regimens.

Generally, people with epilepsy believe doctors could make a greater contribution to its control. Sharing information and making patients coparticipants would not, of course, change its social stigma. This strategy would, however, provide sufferers with more resources in managing epilepsy. Were doctors to better understand the social experience of epilepsy, they might become true allies in the struggle for control and independence.

NINE

The Meaning of
Medications

Drugs have become the technique of choice in much modern medical practice. Moreover, patients themselves *expect* to be given one or another kind of medication as part of effective medical treatment. Studies of placebo effects demonstrate that having these expectations met, even by chemically inert pills, can contribute to a patient's sense of well-being and reduced symptoms. The existence, prescription, and use of medications, then, constitute an integral part of the typical relationships between doctors and patients.

Medication is a particularly important element in the treatment and experience of chronic illnesses such as diabetes, heart disease, and, of course, epilepsy. Considering both the medical and social significance of these chronic illnesses, it is surprising that little sociological research has taken medications, their prescription *and* use, as a topic for study. When it has been studied, it is seen within the context of the doctor-expert/patient-layperson relationship, as something doctors prescribe and patients take. The important questions for study have turned on identifying why patients fail to follow doctors' medication orders. In this chapter, we examine something usually ignored by physicians and others who adopt a medical perspective in their research: what prescribed medications *mean* to the people with epilepsy we interviewed, and how these meanings are reflected in their use.

Prescribing, altering, and monitoring medications to control seizures is the primary if not sole medical management strategy for epilepsy. Given the range of types of epilepsy and the variety of physiological reactions to these medications, patients often see doctors as having a difficult time getting their medications "right." There are starts and stops and changes, depending on the degree of seizure control and the drug's side effects. More often than not, patients are stabilized on a medication or combination at a given dosage or regimen. When there is no change in seizure activity or reaction to medications, routine visits to the doctor mean a brief physical examination, some questions about seizure activity, and a prescription refill.

Medications are important to people with epilepsy because they "control" seizures and because they are a routine part of their everyday lives. Most take these medications several times daily. Although all of our respondents were taking or had taken these drugs, their responses to them varied. The effectiveness of these drugs in controlling seizures is a matter of degree. For some, seizures are stopped completely; they take pills regularly and have no seizures. For most, seizure frequency and duration are decreased significantly, although not reduced to zero. For a very few of our respondents, medications seem to have little impact; seizures continue unabated. The social response to medications—how people define and use these drugs—also varies. Some people take their medications exactly as prescribed, conforming carefully to both the amount and timing of each dose. Others alter their dosage or regimen schedule, or even stop taking their medications altogether.

Nearly all our respondents said medications have helped them at one time or another. This usually meant that they experienced fewer or less severe seizures. At the same time, however, many people changed their dosage and regimen from those medically prescribed. If medications were seen as so helpful, why were nearly half of our respondents "noncompliant" with their doctors' orders?

According to medical culture, patients who follow doctors' orders act properly—they conform to medical rules and are "compliant." Those who refuse or fail to conform represent "problems" or are "difficult" in doctors' eyes (see Lorber, 1975). This medical classification of compliant and noncompliant patients has been used by both physicians and some social scientists in an attempt to understand why some patients deviate from, while others follow medical rules. From the physician's viewpoint, this is a reasonable set of definitions since he or she is concerned with getting the patient to follow medical instructions toward stabilization, improvement, or cure. But from the perspective of the patient the issue may be not at all one of compliance (see Stimson, 1975; Arluke, 1980; Zola, 1981). From the "inside" of illness experience, patterns in *using* medications look quite different.

Most people with illnesses, even chronic illnesses such as epilepsy, spend only a tiny fraction of their lives in the "patient role." Compliance assumes that the doctor-patient relationship is pivotal for subsequent action, which may not be the case. Consistent with our perspective, we conceptualize the issue as one of developing a *medication practice*. Medication practice offers a patient-centered view of how people manage their medications, focusing on the meaning and use of medications. In this light we can see the doctor's medication orders as the "prescribed medication practice" (e.g., take a 20 mg. pill four times a day). Patients interpret the doctor's prescribed regimen and create a medication practice that may vary decidedly from it. Rather than assume the patient will follow prescribed medical rules, this perspective allows us to explore the kinds of practices patients create without couching them in the evaluative terms of compliance or noncompliance. Moreover, whereas compliance/noncompliance is a classification or typology of patients, of persons, our medication practice perspective organizes experience in terms of ways of managing medication; it is a typology of *strategies*. This allows us a considerably broader vantage point for seeing the complexity of how people actually define and use prescribed drugs.

Although many people failed to conform to their prescribed medication regimen, they did not define this conduct primarily as noncompliance with doctors' orders. The more we examined the data, the clearer it was that from the patient's perspective, doctors had very little impact on people's decisions to alter their medications. Rather, it was much more a question of regulation, of control. To examine this more closely we developed criteria for what we could call self-regulation. Many of our respondents occasionally missed taking their medicine, but otherwise were regular in their medication practice. One had to do more than "miss" medications now and again (even a few times a week) to be deemed self-regulating. A person had to (1) reduce or raise the daily dosage of prescribed drugs for several weeks or more, or (2) skip or take extra doses regularly under specific circumstances (e.g., when drinking, staying up late, or coping with "stress"), or (3) stop taking the drugs completely for three consecutive days or longer. These criteria are arbitrary, but they allow us to estimate the extent of self-regulation. Using this definition, thirty-four of our eighty respondents (42 percent) self-regulated their medications.

To understand the meaning and management of medications we need to look at those who follow a prescribed medication practice as well as those who create their own variations. While we note that 42 percent of our respondents are at variance with medical expectations, this number is more suggestive than definitive. Self-regulators are not a discrete and separate group. About half the self-regulators could be defined as regular in their practice, whatever it might be. They may have stopped for a week once or twice, or they may take extra medication only under "stressful" circumstances; otherwise, they are regular in their practice. On the other hand, perhaps a fourth of those following the prescribed medical practice say they have seriously considered changing or stopping their medications. Self-regulating and medical-regulating groups probably overlap. While one needs to appreciate and examine the whole range of medication practice, the self-regulators provide a unique resource for analysis. They articulate views that are probably shared in varying degrees by all people with epilepsy and offer an unusual insight into the meanings of medications and medication practice. We begin by describing how people account for following a prescribed medication practice; we then examine explanations offered for altering prescribed regimens and establishing their own practices. A final section outlines how the meaning of medications constructs and reflects the experience of epilepsy.

A TICKET TO NORMALITY

The discovery of effective seizure control medications early in this century was a milestone in the treatment of epilepsy. These drugs literally changed the experience of having epilepsy. To the extent that the medications controlled seizures, people with epilepsy suffered fewer convulsive disruptions in their lives and were more able to achieve conventional social roles. To the extent that doctors believed the medications effective, they developed greater optimism about their ability to treat epileptic patients. And, to the extent that the public recognized epilepsy as a "treatable" disorder, epileptics were no longer segregated in colonies or subjected as frequently to restrictive laws regarding marriage, procreation, and work. It is not surprising that people with epilepsy regard medications as a "ticket" to normality. The drugs did not, strictly speaking, affect anything but seizures. It was the social response to medication that brought about most of these changes. As one woman said, "I'm glad we've got [the medications]. . . . You know, in the past people didn't and they were looked upon as lepers."

For most people with epilepsy, taking medicine becomes one of those routines of everyday life that we engage in to avoid unwanted circumstances or to improve our health. Respondents compared it to taking vitamins or birth control pills, or brushing their teeth. It becomes almost habitual, something done regularly with little reflection. One young working man said, "Well, at first I didn't like it, [but] it doesn't bother me anymore. Just like getting up in the morning and brushing your teeth. It's just something you do."

But seizure control medications differ from "normal pills" like vitamins or contraceptives. They are prescribed for a medical disorder and are seen, both by the individual and others, as indicators or evidence of having epilepsy. One young man as a child did not know he had epilepsy "short of taking [his] medication." He said of this connection between epilepsy and medications, "I do, so therefore I have." Medications represent epilepsy: Dilantin or phenobarbital are quickly recognized by medical people and often by others as epilepsy medications.

Medications can also indicate the degree of one's disorder. Since most of our respondents do not know any others with epilepsy, they examine changes in their own epilepsy biographies as grounds for conclusions about their condition. Seizure activity is one such sign; the amount of medications "necessary" is another. A decrease or increase in seizures is taken to mean that epilepsy is getting better or worse. So it is with medications. While the two may be related—especially because the common medical response to more seizures is increased medication—they may also operate independently. If the doctor reduces the dose or strength of a medication, or vice versa, the patient may interpret this as a sign of improvement or worsening. Similarly, if a person reduces his or her own dose, being able to "get along" on this lowered amount of medications is taken as evidence of "getting better." Since for a large portion of people with epilepsy seizures are considered to be well-controlled, medications become the only readily available measure of the "progress" of the disorder.

TAKING MEDICATIONS

The reason people gave most often for taking medication is *instrumental*: to control seizures. The medicine is defined as necessary for the body to function properly, or, more to the point, to reduce the likelihood of body malfunction. Our respondents often drew a parallel to the reason people with diabetes take insulin. As one woman said, "If it does the trick, I'd rather take them [medications] than not." Or, as a man who would "absolutely not" miss his medications explained, "I don't want to have seizures" (although he continued to have three or four a month). A former college athlete took his medication because "I know what it's like to be sick." The fear, even terror, for some, of seizures is surely a significant factor, as noted by one woman: "It would scare me . . . not to take it. I would like not to take it but then I guess I would have a real bad one [seizure] again." Those who deal with their medications on instrumental grounds see it simply as a fact of life, as something to be done to avoid body malfunction and social and personal disruption.

While controlling body malfunction is always an underlying reason for taking medications, psychological grounds may be equally compelling. Many people said that taking medication *reduces worry*, independent of its actually decreasing seizures. These drugs can make people feel more secure. A 20-year-old woman remarked: "My pills keep me from getting hysterical." A woman who has taken seizure control medications for fifteen years describes this "psychological" function of medication: "I don't know what it does, but I suppose I'm psychologically dependent on it. In other words, if I take my medication, I feel better." A man who had taken medications for twenty-two years said he worries when he misses:

> A lot of time I think [taking medications is] halfway
> psychological . . . I think it [prevents seizures] be-
> cause I think that I've taken my medicine [so] I'm up
> for it. And I've done this many times. Did I take my
> medicine or didn't I take my medicine and then I
> think, I've taken it. It doesn't affect me, but if I defi-
> nitely know I didn't and I forgot it and I'm some-
> where I don't have any medicine, it starts to irri-
> tate [me].

Some people actually report "feeling better"—clearer, more alert and energetic—when they do not take these drugs, but because they begin to worry if they miss, they take them regularly anyway.

The most important reason for taking medications, however, is to insure "normality." People said specifically that they take medications to be more "normal": "medications make me normal" or "it is something I do to be normal." The meaning here is normal in the sense of "leading a normal life." A middle-aged public relations executive said that he does not restrict his life because of epilepsy but that he always takes his medications. He continued, "I don't know why. I figure if I took them, then I could do anything I wanted to do." People believed taking medicine reduces the risk of having a seizure in the presence of others, which might be embarrassing or frightening. As a young woman explained: "I feel if it's going to help, that's what I want because you know you feel uncomfortable enough anyway that you don't want anything like that [a seizure] to happen around other people; so if it's going to help, I'll take it." But a sense of having to take medication as a prophylactic against social disruption can engender resentment. A man in his early twenties commented: "Just the thought that you're going to have to go through the rest of your life taking little pills, so you don't have a fit in front of somebody and scare them to death, that bugs me." The social risks of not taking medication can be high, especially of upsetting the delicate balance of normal appearances. Thus, people are hesitant to "gamble," "take chances," or "look for trouble" because they "can't afford the problems if they miss and have a bad seizure."

This is not to say people with epilepsy like to take medications. Quite the contrary. Many respondents who follow their medically prescribed medication practice openly say that they "hate" taking medications and hope someday to be "off" them. Part of this distaste is related to the dependence people come to feel. Some used the metaphor of being an addict: "I'm a real drug addict"; "I was an addict before it was fashionable"; "I'm like an alcoholic without a drink; I *have* to have them [pills]"; and "I really don't want to be hooked for the rest of my life." Even while loathing the pills or the "addiction," people may be quite disciplined about taking these drugs. In their own terms, they "never miss." But the reasons or accounts they give have more to do with the meanings of their medications for them than with the authority of the doctor's orders.

The drugs used to control seizures are not, of course, foolproof. Some people continue to have seizures quite regularly while others suffer only occasional episodes. Such limited effectiveness does not necessarily lead these people to reject medication as a strategy. They continue, with frustration, to express "hope" that "they [doctors] will get it [the medication] right." For some, then, medications are but a limited ticket to normality.

SELF-REGULATION: GROUNDS FOR CHANGING MEDICATION PRACTICE

For most people there is not a one-to-one correspondence between taking or missing medications and seizure activity. People who take medications regularly may still have seizures, and some people who discontinue their medications may be seizure-free for months or longer. Medical experts say a patient may well miss a whole day's medication yet still have enough of the drug in the bloodstream to prevent a seizure for this period.

In this section we focus on those who deviate from the prescribed medication practice and variously regulate their own medications. On the whole, members of this subgroup are slightly younger than the rest of the sample (average age of twenty-five versus thirty-two) and somewhat more likely to be female (59 percent to 43 percent), but otherwise are not remarkably different from our respondents who follow the prescribed medication practice. Self-regulation for most of our respondents consists of reducing the dosage, stopping for a time, or regularly skipping or taking extra doses of medication depending on various circumstances. For the purpose of this analysis we will consider all these to be forms of self-regulation.

Reducing the dosage (including total termination) is the most common form of self-regulation. In this context, two points are worth restating. First, doctors typically alter dosage of medication in times of increased seizure activity or troublesome drug "side effects." It is difficult to strike the optimum level of medication. To people with epilepsy, it seems that doctors engage in a certain amount of trial and error behavior. Second, and more important, medications are defined, both by doctors and patients, as an indicator of the degree of disorder. If seizure activity is not "controlled," or increases, patients see that doctors respond by raising (or changing) medications. What doctors do does not necessarily explain what patients do, but it may well be an example our respondents use in their own management strategies.

The efficacy of a drug is a complex issue. Here our concern is merely with perceived efficacy. When a medication is no longer *seen* as efficacious it is likely to be stopped. Many people continue to have seizures even when they follow the prescribed medication practice. If medication seemed to make no difference, our respondents were more likely to consider changing their medication practice. One woman who stopped taking medications for a couple of months said, "It seemed like [I had] the same number of seizures without it." Having to take medication with no marked seizure reduction made this young man angry:

> When I was young . . . I just rebelled against the whole damn thing. I said, the hell with it, I don't want it. You can take your medicine and go to hell. I just said I can cut back—I can whip this on my own, but every time I tried it I just kept having seizures and, uh, I was still having the seizures with the medicine. That's what made me mad. . . . I was probably having an average of five a week. . . . it was not cutting them out completely and that was what pissed me off. And as I say, if I got to take these things they better work. It wasn't one hundred percent and I threw it out several times, and then went back to it, of course.

Most people who stop taking their medicine altogether eventually resume a medication practice of some sort. A woman college instructor said, "When I was taking Dilantin, I stopped a number of times because it never seemed to *do* anything." We asked why she always went back to the medications. She replied:

> Each time the doctor would say it would make a difference and I guess you wanna be liked, so [the] doctor says "Do this" [and I do]. I really don't know why because . . . again supposedly they know something you don't. You pay them thirty dollars and they say, "Put this little thing in your *mouth*." And you know, maybe it has something to do with getting your money's worth.

Both figuratively and literally, if patients believe the prescribed medication practice does not "give them their money's worth," they consider changing it.

The most common drug-related rationale for reducing dosage is troublesome side effects (we adopt the term side effects here in its common medical usage, because this is how our respondents use it; clearly what a "side effect" is is dependent on what the "main" effect is defined to be). People with epilepsy attribute a variety of side effects to seizure control medications. One category of effects includes swollen and bleeding gums, oily or yellow skin, pimples, sore throat and a rash. Another category includes slowed mental functioning, drowsiness, slurred speech, dullness, impaired memory, loss of balance and partial impotence.* The first category, which we can call body side effects, were virtually never given as an account for self-regulation. Only those side effects that impaired social skills, those in the second category, were given as reasons for altering doctors' medication orders. If people saw their medication practice as hindering the ability to participate in routine social affairs, they were likely to change it. Our respondents gave a number of examples. A self-regulating woman described how she feels when she takes her medi-

---

* These are *reported* side effects. They may or may not be drug related, but our respondents attribute them to the medication.

cation: "I can feel that I become much more even. I feel like I flatten out a little bit. I don't like that feeling. . . . It's just a feeling of dullness, which I don't like, almost a feeling that you're on the edge of laziness." A college student claimed the medication slowed him down. He wondered if it was affecting his memory. A young newspaper reporter reduced his medication when he said it was putting him to sleep at work. A young social worker decreased her medication and finally stopped altogether, because she feels "more alert, more articulate" and does not "talk so slow" as when she was taking the medication. She felt she "sounded smarter" when she was "off medications." One woman who stopped her medications entirely contended she would rather suffer one or two seizures a month (which came conveniently early in the morning) than take medication that made her feel constantly drowsy and disconnected from her environment.

Drug side effects, even those that impair social skills, are not sufficient in themselves to explain the level of self-regulation we found. Self-regulation was considerably more than a reaction to annoying and uncomfortable side effects. It was an active and intentional endeavor.

SOCIAL MEANINGS OF REGULATING MEDICATION PRACTICE

Variations in medication practice by and large seem to depend on what medication and self-regulation mean to our respondents. Troublesome relationships with physicians, including the perception that they have provided inadequate medical information (Korsch et al., 1968), may encourage alternative strategies and practices. Our respondents, however, did not cite such grounds for altering their doctors' orders. Their reasons were connected more to managing their everyday lives. If we examine the social meanings of medications from our respondents' perspectives, self-regulation turns on four grounds: testing; control of dependence; destigmatization; and practical practice.

TESTING

According to our respondents, once they began taking seizure-control medications doctors seldom changed the medical regimen unless there were special problems or seizures. People are likely to stay on medications indefinitely. The assumption is, of course, that epilepsy is a chronic illness and that sufferers will need medications throughout their lives (at least if seizures persist past childhood). But how can one know whether a period without seizures is a result of medication or a spontaneous remission of the disorder? How long can one go without medication? How "bad" is this case of epilepsy? How can one know if epilepsy is "getting better" while still taking medication? Frequently, after a period without or with only a few seizures, people reduced or stopped their medicine altogether to test for themselves whether or not epilepsy was "still there."

People can take themselves off medications as an experiment, to see "if anything will happen." One woman recalled: "I was having one to two seizures a year on phenobarb . . . so I decided not to take it and to see what would happen . . . so I stopped it and I watched and it seemed that I had the same amount of seizures with it as without it . . . for three years." She told her physician, who was skeptical but "allowed" her this control of her medication practice. A man who had taken medication three times a day for sixteen years felt intuitively that he could stop his medications: "Something kept telling me I didn't have to take [medication] anymore, a feeling or somethin'. It took me quite a while to work up the nerve to stop takin' the pills. And one day I said, 'One way to find out . . .'" After suffering what he called drug withdrawal effects, he had no seizures for six years. Others test to see how long they can go without medications and seizures.

Testing does not always turn out successfully. A public service agency executive tried twice to stop taking medications when he thought he had "kicked" epilepsy. After two failures, he concluded that stopping medications "just doesn't work":

Yes, I did change my medication. I was on one . . . 100 mg. capsule from 1960 'til 1964 and I had not had a seizure in that form for a five-year period with one capsule, so I went to a doctor and I said, "Hey, you know, I've kicked it." [laughs] "Maybe so." So I was off medication for a period of time and then had another seizure and I says, "Uh-oh. Didn't kick it. Still got it." So then I went back to one capsule, 100 mg. Dilantin capsule a day from then until about 1972 . . . and I got to the point, well I hadn't had a seizure for another five to seven years. It was a long period of time. No seizure, I kicked it. So, I got sloppy. I didn't take my medication and I missed it for three or four days or whatever and I had a small seizure at home and I said, "Uh-oh, shape up," and in fact, I got religion, you might say. I increased my medication.

But others continued to test, hoping for some change in their condition. One middle-aged housewife said:

When I was young I would try not to take it. . . . I'd take it for a while and think, "Well, I don't need it anymore," so I would not take it for, deliberately, just to see if I could do without. And then [in a few days] I'd start takin' it again, because I'd start passin' out. . . . I will still try that now, when my husband is out of town. . . . I just think, maybe I'm still gonna grow out of it or something.

Occasionally people test as a result of a specific experience. Two of our respondents felt they had been "healed by the Lord" at a healing ceremony and stopped taking their medication. Both had seizures within three days and began taking the drug again. Testing by reducing or stopping medication is only one way to evaluate how one's disorder is progressing. Even respondents who follow the prescribed medication regimen often wonder "just what would happen" if they stopped.

CONTROLLING DEPENDENCE

People with epilepsy struggle continually against becoming too dependent on family, friends, doctors, or medications. They do, of course, depend on medications for control of seizures. The medications do not necessarily eliminate seizures and many of our respondents resented their dependence on them. Another paradox is that although medications can increase self reliance by reducing seizures, taking medications can be *experienced* as a threat to self reliance. Medications seem almost to become symbolic of the dependence created by having epilepsy.

There is a widespread belief in our society that drugs create dependence and that being dependent on chemical substances is not a good thing. Somehow, whatever the goal is, it is thought to be better if we can get there without drugs. Our respondents reflected these ideas in their comments.

A college junior explained, "I don't like it at all. I don't like chemicals in my body. It's sort of like a dependency only that I have to take it because my body forced me to. . . ." A political organizer who says medications reduce his seizures commented, "I've never enjoyed having to depend on anything . . . drugs in particular." A nurse summed up the situation: "The *drugs* were really a kind of dependence."

Some said although the medications controlled seizures they felt they themselves did not control the drug. It was as if the drug were controlling them. The political organizer continued, "Primarily it's a minor irritation that I have to take drugs every day." We asked why he took LSD as a recreational drug but disliked epilepsy medications. He said:

I mind having to be . . . controlled by them to a certain extent, that's what I really mind about it. Those
other things I did for a certain enjoyment. . . . I just,
uh, y'know, don't like to have, y'know, things com-
manding me so much, and so on, that's all.

A woman said:

I don't like to have to *take* anything. It was, like, at
one time birth control pills, but I don't like to take
anything *every day*. It's just like, y'know, controlling
me, or something. I don't like the idea of having to do
that. . . . I have to tell myself that, and nobody's telling
me that, but I just have that feeling. But I do take it.
And I don't miss very often.

The feeling of being controlled need not be substantiated
in fact for people to act upon it. If people *feel* dependent
on and controlled by medication, it is not surprising that
they seek to avoid these drugs. A high school junior, who
once took medicine because he feared having a seizure in
the street, commented, "And I'd always heard medicine
helps and I just kept taking it and finally I just got so I
didn't depend on the medicine no more, I could just fight
it off myself and I just stopped taking it in." After stopping
for a month he forgot about his medications completely.

Feelings of dependence are one reason people gave for
regulating medication. For a year, one young social worker
took medication when she felt it was necessary; otherwise,
she tried not to use it. When we asked her why, she responded, "I regulate my own drug . . . mostly because it's
really important for me not to be dependent." She occasionally had seizures and continued to alter her medication to try to "get it right":

I started having [seizures] every once in a while. And I
thought wow, the bad thing is that I just haven't regulated it right and I just need to up it a little bit and
then, you know, if I do it just right, I won't have epilepsy anymore.

This woman and others saw medications as a powerful tool

in their struggle to gain control over epilepsy. Although she no longer thinks she can rid herself of epilepsy, this woman still regulates her medication.

People with epilepsy sometimes feel that family or friends increase their dependence on medications. Some reported that they regulated their medication intake in direct response to interventions of others, especially family members who coaxed or reminded them to take their medications regularly. They felt as if others wanted them to be more dependent. Many responded to this by creating their own medication practices.

A housewife who said she continues regularly to have petit mal seizures and tremors along with an occasional grand mal seizure, remarked:

> Oh, like most things, when someone tells me I have to do something, I basically resent it. . . . If it's my option and I choose to do it, I'll probably do it more often than not. But if you tell me I have to, I'll bend it around and do it my own way, which is basically what I have done.

One man, an actor, felt he was being manipulated by his family. He recalled stopping taking medication in response.

> One time, yes, when I was a freshman in college. I stopped taking it for a couple of days . . . because at the time I was thinking, I don't need to do this. But now I realize I was obviously tempting myself. . . . I suppose if I . . . could stop takin' that and not have seizures . . . that would be proof I was being manipulated.

We asked him to whom this would be "proof":

> My family. . . . . I found an old poem I once wrote about being poisoned. . . . It goes, "Asking your opinion, I received a pill, It should have poisoned me but I outfoxed you, claiming to be ill."

Because he felt manipulated he manipulated his medication practice to assert some degree of autonomy. In a similar vein, a woman who defines herself as "a very independent person" decided she no longer wanted to take her medication. She was convinced by her family and doctor to try again. Rather than simply telling her to follow the prescribed practice, they included her in the decision making: "They aren't at this point saying 'You take that.' They are *suggesting* it to me, which I feel much better about. . . . You know, they are giving me the decision." This coparticipant stance has encouraged her even to consider taking a newly available drug.

Whether one feels dependent on the drug or on others who intervene to encourage drug taking, self-regulation serves as a form of *taking control* of one's epilepsy.

DESTIGMATIZATION

As we discussed earlier, epilepsy is a stigmatized illness. Sufferers attempt to control information about the disorder to manage this threat. There are no visible stigmata that make a person with epilepsy obviously different from other people, but a number of aspects of having epilepsy can compromise attempts at information control. The four signs that our respondents most frequently mentioned as threatening information control were seizures in the presence of others, job or insurance applications, lack of a driver's license, and use of medications. People may try to avoid seizures in public, lie or hedge on their applications, develop accounts for not having a driver's license, or take their medicine in private in order to minimize the stigma potential of epilepsy.

Medication usually must be taken three or four times daily, so at least one dose must be taken away from home. People attempt to be private about taking their medications and/or develop "normal" pill accounts ("it's to help my digestion."). One woman's mother told her to take her medications regularly, as she would for any other sickness: "When I was younger it didn't bother me too bad. But as I got older, it would tend to bother me some. Whether it was, y'know, maybe somebody seeing me or somethin', I don't know. But it did." A recent high school graduate was concerned that other students would wonder why he was taking pills:

> The only time it bothers me is when I have to take it and I'm not at home. When I was at school I had to have the bottle sitting in my locker so I could take it at noon. And you sit there [by] your locker and they say "What's this . . . popping pills?"

Most people develop skills to minimize potential stigmatization from taking pills in public.

On occasion, people simply stop taking medications in an attempt to avoid the stigmatized status of epileptic. One respondent wrote us a letter describing how she tried to get her mother to accept her by not taking her medications. She wrote:

> This is going to sound real dumb, but I can't help it. My mother never accepted me when I was little because I was "different." I stopped taking my medication in an attempt to be normal and accepted by her. Now that I know I need medication it's like I'm completely giving up trying to be "normal" so mom won't be ashamed of me. I'm going to accept the fact that I'm "different" and I don't really care if mom gives a damn or not.

Taking medications is in effect an acknowledgment of this "differentness."

It is, of course, more difficult to hide the meaning of medications from one's self. Taking medication is a constant reminder of having epilepsy. For some it is as if the medication itself represents the stigma of epilepsy. The young social worker felt that if she could stop taking her medications, she would no longer be an epileptic. Asked how she felt about taking her medications, a young woman hospital technician replied:

> I resent it. . . . Sometimes on days when I'm more depressed or something like that it takes me an awful

long time to take them 'cuz they'll just sit there in front of me and I'll look at them and think of all the kooks that are out there purposely taking pills and here I have to take them. I just resent the whole fact. At one point she stopped taking her medications. She said, "A couple of years ago I did 'cuz when I refused to accept I had epilepsy I don't know what I was thinking. I suppose I thought if I didn't take my pills it would go away, but it didn't, it just got worse." A young working woman summed up succinctly why avoiding medications would be avoiding stigma: "Well, at least I would not be . . . generalized and classified in a group as being an epileptic."

PRACTICAL PRACTICE

Self-regulators spoke often of how they changed the dose or regimen of medication in an effort to reduce the risk of having a seizure, particularly during "high stress" situations. Several respondents who were students said that they take extra medications during exam periods or when they stay up late studying. A law student who had not taken his medicine for six months took some before his law school exams: "I think it increases the chances [seizures] won't happen." A woman who often participated in horse shows said she "usually didn't pay attention" to her medication practice but takes extra when she doesn't get the six to eight hours sleep she requires: "I'll wake up and take two capsules instead of one . . . and I'll generally take it like when we're going to horse shows. I'll take it pretty consistently." Such uses of medication are common ways of trying to forestall "possible trouble." One woman who was already on a high dosage of medication said, "When I'm having trouble, I add another 250 milligrams [of Mysoline]." These extra doses were a kind of added insurance against seizures.

People with epilepsy changed their medication practice for practical ends in two other kinds of circumstances.

Several reported they took extra medication if they felt a "tightening" or felt a seizure coming on. Many people also said they did not take medications if they were going to drink alcohol. They believed that medication (especially phenobarbital) and alcohol do not mix well. A woman explained:

> Like I say, when I know it's . . . like a New Year's eve or if we're going on a Jaycee convention or somethin' . . . I'll take some before we go . . . but then, well if it's a three day weekend like on Saturday I won't because I know I'm . . . drinking and stuff. Then, I'll still take my Dilantin but I will not take the phenobarbital if I'm gonna drink.

In short, people change their medication practice to suit their perceptions of social environment. Some reduce medication to avoid potential problems from mixing alcohol and drugs. Others reduce it to remain "clear-headed" and "alert" during "important" performances (something of a "Catch-22" situation). Most, however, adjust their medications practically in an effort to reduce the risk of seizures.

ASSERTING CONTROL

Regulating medication represents an attempt to assert some degree of control over a condition that appears at times to be completely beyond control. Loss of control is a significant concern for people with epilepsy. While medical treatment can increase both the sense and fact of control over epilepsy, and information control can limit stigmatization, the regulation of medications is one way people with epilepsy struggle to gain some personal control over their condition.

Medication practice can be modified on several different grounds. Side effects that make managing everyday social interaction difficult can lead to the reduction or termination of medication. People will change their medication practice, including stopping altogether, in order to "test" for the existence or "progress" of the disorder. Medication may be altered to control the perceived level of dependence, either on the drugs themselves or on those who "push" them to adhere to a particular medication practice. Since the medication can represent the stigma potential of epilepsy, both literally and symbolically, altering medication practice is for some a form of destigmatization. And finally, many people modify their medication practice in anticipation of specific social circumstances, usually attempting to reduce the risk of seizures.

A large proportion of the people with epilepsy we interviewed said they themselves regulate their medication. From the perspective of the person with epilepsy, the issue is more clearly one of responding to the meaning of medications in everyday life than of "compliance" with physicians' orders and medical regimens.

TEN

Having Epilepsy: The Experience and Control of Illness

We cannot understand illness experience by studying disease alone, for disease refers merely to undesirable changes in the body. Illness, however, is primarily about social meanings, experiences, relationships, and conduct that exist around putative disease. People may have diseases without being ill, and vice versa.* Physicians and medical science are the official man-

---

*The former is problematic in that we do not know that a person has a disease until he or she has been diagnosed. Since diagnosis usually is done by medical professionals, to be deemed "diseased" by a doctor is to become officially recognized as ill. As for illness without disease, some critics of modern psychiatry (Szasz, 1970; Torrey, 1973) hold that "mental illness" is precisely such a case.

agers of disease (on balance, for our own good fortune). We have tried to examine having epilepsy as a social experience and process that occurs, for the most part, outside the scrutiny of professional medicine. This nonprofessional/ noninstitutional context is particularly important to people living with chronic illnesses, including epilepsy.

Our respondents spent considerable time with epilepsy as something they (rather than doctors) managed and attempted to control. Although there were people who seemed not to struggle against *both* disorder and illness, who in effect "gave up" and became debilitated, most directly pursued adaptations to live more normal lives (see Schneider and Conrad, 1981).

Research on the experience of chronic illness has begun to show us that people *can* understand this experience without relying entirely on medical experts. People with illnesses act on these sometimes more or less correct understandings to care for themselves in a variety of commonplace, everyday ways. The important care that people give themselves seems to go unnoticed by both them and most students of illness. We as laypersons have given up almost completely the idea that these homely things we do for ourselves are therapeutic, that they do constitute care. It has been given up in an historical process through which professional medicine has gained an almost complete monopoly on control of body/mind problems. Efficacy aside, as medicine has taken more control, including the prerogatives even to define what is happening, people with illnesses themselves seem to experience less (see Comaroff and Maguire, 1981).

But people do take responsibility not only for monitoring their diseases and illnesses, but also for managing them. They do this for the sense of control they gain as well as for the practical benefits (e.g., stabilized or improved illness trajectories). We argue later in this chapter that if people better appreciated the central part they play in the dramas of their own health and illness they could then exert a

more systematically positive influence than they sometimes do.

In this last chapter we attempt to place what we learned
about the experience of epilepsy within the more general
context of illness experience. We close the chapter with
suggestions for change.

ILLNESS AND EPILEPSY: GENERAL CONCERNS AND PARTICULAR INSIGHTS

The closest thing we have to a general framework for
studying illness experience is Strauss and Glaser's (1975)
book on "chronic illness and the quality of life." They identify major issues people face as they live their lives with
and in spite of their conditions. We forge their ideas with
our own in the following discussion.

MANAGING UNCERTAINTY

A defining quality of most chronic conditions is uncertainty. From the first "signs of trouble," through diagnosis
and discovery, to, for many disorders, their termination in
death, people with these conditions have a great many
questions (most of which remain unasked). They wonder
what is happening to them in their bodies and/or minds;
what their disease or disorder is—the name for which they
may at first recognize only vaguely; how and why they
have it; what its course or trajectory will be; what will happen when; how they will recognize these changes; and
what they mean. They begin to wonder, often while still
recovering in the hospital, how their illness will affect
their future lives and relationships. These and similar questions arise not only in the pre—discovery-and-diagnosis period, but recur in various forms throughout the experience
of illness (see Locker, 1981).

For some illnesses, discovery and diagnosis are drawn

out over considerable time. To many of our respondents, doctors seemed to proceed by trial and error to decide finally what was wrong. In the prediscovery period, our respondents did what many people do when they first notice unusual feelings and body/mind events: they attempt (usually successfully) to see them as inconsequential or familiar—in short, as "normal" (cf. Davis, 1973; Cowie, 1976; Stewart and Sullivan, 1982; Waddell, 1982; Speedling, 1982).

But if the unusual feelings persist, or become severe, people are likely to put aside these strategies for a definition of possible seriousness. A grand mal seizure, a heart attack, persistent fatigue, nausea, or soreness make discounting and "working around" ineffective as strategies. Moreover, these persistent and more serious feelings intrude on everyday activities. People then go or are taken to doctors to find out what is wrong. Sometimes their uncertainty is reduced; sometimes it is not.

Persistent uncertainty, coupled with continuing episodes of trouble and vague information from doctors, led some respondents to construct pessimistic definitions of their condition and fate. They feared the worst, namely a brain tumor or blood clot. Some said they became desperate. One woman tried to commit suicide; another was considering it. David Stewart and Thomas Sullivan (1982) suggest that multiple sclerosis patients actually suffered iatrogenic stress-related disorders due to long periods of uncertainty over their diagnosis. In a study of cystic fibrosis networks, made up mostly of parents, Charles Waddell (1982) found a rather elaborate system of neutralization to keep "faith and hope" alive by deflecting various uncertainties associated with this condition. People do manage uncertainty to minimize their sense of disorder and anxiety, but their resourcefulness is not unlimited.

Our respondents faced uncertainty after diagnosis too, as did Edward Speedling's (1982) heart attack victims. In the case of epilepsy, respondents worried about the possibility of a seizure in some public or "important" place, and about others finding out. Such chronic uncertainty is particularly likely for those with progressive or degenerative diseases, such as rheumatoid arthritis, arteriosclerosis, cancer, diabetes, cystic fibrosis, and muscular dystrophy (see Wiener, 1975; Bluebond-Langner, 1978; Comaroff and Maguire, 1981; Waddell, 1982).

This uncertainty turns not only on the disease process, but on illness as a social and psychological phenomenon. Many questions arise, including how much a person can do without precipitating a medical crisis or more severe symptoms, whether or not certain activities help or exacerbate the disorder, and what the doctor's instructions about daily routine actually mean in terms of specific activities. How to manage established relationships that have been changed suddenly by one's illness, when to think about going back to work, and whether one's relationships with work associates will be "different" are other concerns. And for many with chronic illnesses, there is the ultimate uncertainty of sudden or imminent death. To suffer chronic illness is to live with all of these questions, in varying forms. People deal with this uncertainty; for most it is never far from their thoughts.

KNOWLEDGE OF DISEASE AND ILLNESS AS A RESOURCE

One basis for the uncertainty surrounding chronic illness is a sense of not really understanding the disorder itself. None of the people we interviewed said they knew as much as they wanted to about epilepsy or their own condition. Many said their knowledge of epilepsy consisted of what doctors told them: epilepsy was "like an electrical storm in my brain;" they should take their medication to control seizures, and they should call if they noticed any dramatic changes.

Lay knowledge of disease by and large reflects medical

knowledge. Educational programs offered by various health agencies devoted to specific diseases, such as The Epilepsy Foundation of America, The American Cancer Society, and The Muscular Dystrophy Association are another source of general medical knowledge. People expect their doctors to provide them with specific information about what is happening to *them*. The people we interviewed felt their physicians told them all too little. As a result, they often expressed dissatisfaction with their medical care. In fact, this issue of information sharing between physician and patient was one of the major "problems" people said characterized their relationships with doctors (cf. P. West, 1982; Speedling, 1982; Stewart and Sullivan, 1982). Such information can be an important resource for people in their attempt to manage illness and maintain some sense of mastery in lives threatened with dependence.

Respondents often turned to other sources, including folk wisdom, accounts by friends or family members suffering similar conditions, popular writings about various diseases and illnesses, and in some cases where their education and experience would permit, published medical sources (cf. Stewart and Sullivan, 1982; Comaroff and Maguire, 1981). This "research" activity produced results that were not always accurate and, when turned into action, sometimes made coping with epilepsy more rather than less difficult. This aside, the assertive act of looking for and gaining knowledge about their illness allowed people to *do something* rather than nothing, and thus to reduce their sense of dependence on others (particularly, in this case, physicians).* There were, of course, people who said

---

*Jean Comaroff and Peter Maguire (1981) suggest that as medical technology and control advance, lay people's sense of efficaciousness around their diseases and illnesses decline. It may be that for those diseases and disorders where medicine is most mundane and least technologically sophisticated, such as epilepsy, lay participation in understanding and self care can emerge more completely.

they did not know where to find out about epilepsy except from their doctors. This sense of ignorance about something that was such a part of themselves contributed to a feeling of dependency and lack of control.

RELATIONSHIPS WITH MEDICAL PROFESSIONALS

There is no question that a significant segment of illness experience involves relationships with physicians and other medical personnel, often in hospitals. Extant research on illness has concentrated on the experience of patienthood and hospitalization to the exclusion of other parts of the whole. Future research should continue to show us these institutionalized features of illness experience through the eyes of patients. We need to know more about how physicians, hospitals, and nurses look to those who seek and receive their services.

In this perspective, it is less important to know what doctors actually do than how they appeared to their patients (and families, see Suczek et al., 1982; Speedling, 1982). On balance, our respondents' view of physicians was ambivalent. People with epilepsy need physicians to tell them what is wrong, to prescribe an effective course of treatment, to monitor medication levels and effectiveness, and to provide information about their condition. They must (and some want to) depend on their physicians. At the same time, however, many spoke of being dissatisfied with the effectiveness of the treatment and with their personal rapport with doctors (cf. Stewart and Sullivan, 1982).

Another study of people with epilepsy (Wallace, 1982) found that of all others they routinely encountered, respondents had the highest expectations for physicians. The gap between people's expectations and their experience may explain some of this dissatisfaction. Moreover, the effect of medical care for chronic illnesses is much more one of containment and control than cure. At the same time, we have no reason to doubt what our respondents told us about the details of their medical care. Since most research on the doctor-patient relationship has minimized the patient's viewpoint, we have a one-sided understanding of the problems that define health care delivery.

Perceptions of doctors as "brusque," "routine," "very businesslike," "cold," uncommunicative (see P. West, 1982), and sometimes unknowledgeable in treating epilepsy (cf. Hopkins and Scambler, 1977; Beran et al., 1981) left many respondents with mixed feelings about physicians. People with chronic diseases need doctors. Research on the experience of illness must address more precisely the patterns, peculiarities, and contexts that define these relationships.

MANAGING REGIMENS

The word "regimen" evokes first and foremost the idea of medical prescription: things doctors tell patients to do to stabilize or improve their conditions. Studies of medical regimen have focused on the issue of compliance, usually attempting to understand the patient's *lack* of compliance with doctor's orders. Approaching the issue of regimen this way leads us to questions about the forms and shapes of noncompliance and ways to encourage conformity. It paints this kind of patient behavior in one moral hue: "bad." Yet this is only part of the story of managing regimens. Experience-of-illness research must not adopt medical prescription as its point of departure. What is compliance and noncompliance from the doctor's viewpoint most assuredly is something else to the person with the illness.

Even when patients do conform to medical regimens, it is probably more accurate to speak of this as a managed accomplishment. It is the patient who must put the (sometimes vague) rules into practice. Some of our respondents, for instance, were very regular in taking medication, but not without *working* at it. They devised a variety of strategies to remember to take this or that medication at the correct time of day, each day. The fact that such drug-taking becomes routine does not mean it happens "automatically" or outside one's consciousness.

People managed their medication in another way that turns the issue of compliance on its head. Almost half of the people we interviewed altered the medication regimen prescribed by their doctors. More significantly, they established one of their own. While virtually all alternated between this and the prescribed practice, occasionally negotiating dosage with their doctors, taking charge of medication regimen was a common feature of the experience of epilepsy.

Managing regimens, then, is not only about following medical rules. While people still took drugs, they nevertheless established patterns based on 1) their own sense of seizure experience, 2) the perceived effectiveness of the drug, 3) the presence of undesirable side effects, 4) the desire to test to see if their epilepsy was "still there," 5) the wish to avoid having others (and perhaps themselves) recognize they had epilepsy, and 6) the need to insure against seizures in difficult situations. Independent of the medical wisdom of such management, taking control of medication meant taking some control of epilepsy and themselves. Edward Speedling (1982) studied eight families in which the husband-father suffered a heart attack. These men, their spouses, and children maintained almost complete control over regimen (not without conflict). People with diabetes (Benoliel, 1975) and their significant others are quite clearly in charge of both diet and insulin regimens. Those with ulcerative colitis must devote much time and energy to pollution control (Reif, 1975). Most chronic conditions require a good deal of management work by those afflicted (see Strauss and Glaser, 1975).

SYMPTOM AND CRISIS
CONTROL

According to convention, physicians are thought responsible for controlling the symptoms of disease and disorder. If patients follow doctors' orders symptoms should be controlled. The problem, as noted, is to convince people they should do what doctors say. Such a view is both simplistic and incomplete.

Physicians do provide regimens to control symptoms and/or disease. Physicians' knowledge, however, is grounded primarily in an understanding of the general case, the *type* of disease or disorder and its typical symptoms and course. It is with the patient that the individual variations emerge. In addition, physicians' knowledge is largely external and professional. People with diseases and disorders have another kind of knowledge. They know their symptoms in a way that doctors and others cannot. The ill can *experience* the symptoms directly. This most fundamental fact of disease and disorder potentially provides the sufferer with grounds for a detailed, highly specific knowledge of his or her body. Physicians necessarily rely on such patient-provided knowledge for diagnosis and treatment, particularly for disorders such as epilepsy (cf. Stewart and Sullivan, 1982).

Sensitivity to one's symptoms is vital for disorders where symptom occurrence, the disease process, and illness are connected. Cancer and diabetes are examples in which to control symptoms may be also to control disease and illness trajectory. With cancer, symptom control may take the ill person back to medical professionals for chemotherapy or other technologies; for diabetes, it may mean watching diet more closely. The connection between seizures and trajectory for people with epilepsy is less clear. Our respondents, nevertheless, saw seizures as unhappy reminders that their condition was still there. An increase in seizures or an emergence of a more serious type meant that their epilepsy was getting worse. Seizures were also seen as sure evidence of one's affliction.

Ill people can take an active role in managing their own symptoms. Most illness takes place and persists in everyday settings. When they recognize symptoms (and our respondents had to *learn* to recognize them), they can put the professional regimens into practice or call upon alternative, nonprofessional strategies of control. Our respondents invested much time and energy in making special plans "in case" they had a seizure in some public place. Marcella Davis (1973) describes how her respondents with multiple sclerosis "mapped out the environment" before going places to avoid difficult terrain and to insure that a toilet was near at hand.

Symptom control for people with epilepsy means seizure control, but not necessarily by professional regimens alone. Some of our respondents used meditation, biofeedback, specific diets, vitamin supplements, relaxation, altered social plans, and "self control" to stave off seizures. While most people continued to rely on medications, they believed on balance these alternative strategies were also effective (see also, Center for Urban Affairs and Policy Research, n.d.). We need to pay closer attention to the ways people attempt to manage symptoms by using strategies outside professional medicine. These make up part of the lay- or ethno-medicine that students of illness have generally ignored.

FAMILY RELATIONSHIPS

Family relationships, given some degree of competent medical care, are probably the most important of all relationships surrounding the experience of chronic illness. There are exceptions, and physicians are at certain times far more important to the ill than any family member. These ties nevertheless are central features of illness experience. We often miss their significance because we know so little about how illness fits into everyday life. Even our study of epilepsy cannot do full justice to this topic, since we have only our respondents' perceptions of certain key family members (but see Speedling, 1982, and the research on parents of chronically ill children, e.g., Davis, 1963; Bluebond-Langner, 1978; Voysey, 1975; Comaroff and Maguire, 1981; Ziegler, 1981; Waddell, 1982).

Many people told us of complex and contradictory feelings, similar to the ambivalence they felt for doctors, toward family members, particularly parents. Appreciation and resentment, attraction and repulsion, dependence and strongly asserted independence were often recalled simultaneously.

Parents are uniquely important in helping shape their children's perception of the world and of themselves. Some respondents said that their parents conveyed almost apocalyptic definitions of epilepsy and its significance, and then refused to talk about it with them. One mother told her daughter that epilepsy "is something we just don't talk about." It was something disgraceful, to be hidden and denied—quite literally, not to be spoken about. Such definitions made epilepsy a great burden for these children as they grew up. They were likely to conceal it and suffer shame. Other parents were considerably more open, defining epilepsy as a "normal medical problem" that could be handled through medication and a balanced lifestyle. It was not grounds for shame or disgrace. Respondents whose parents adopted this approach commented on the importance of being able to talk about their epilepsy openly. They held definitions of epilepsy to be considerably less significant to their lives and selves.

Parental worry and protection were common problems. Respondents expected parents to "care" about and "look out" for them, but even open and helpful parents could be too concerned about epilepsy. People sometimes spoke about being treated like or feeling like "babies" around their parents. For them, this sense of infantilization (cf. Zola, 1982a) remained strong into adulthood. Their parents often seemed to have an investment in maintaining the asymmetric relationship between themselves and their children that illness transforms and reproduces. This is precisely what Speedling (1982) found between some husbands and wives after a heart attack, where wives actually *thrived* on their husband's dependence.

Our respondents wanted the love, support and attention of family members, and even wanted to be dependent on them—up to a point. The distinction of parents who "made things worse" from those who "helped me deal with it" seemed to turn on a delicate balance between the liberating and controlling effects of caregiving. We know very little about how illness experience is mediated by these family ties (see Corbin and Strauss, 1982).

FRIENDS AND ASSOCIATES

We know almost nothing about how illness is managed in relationships with friends, associates, and in various public interactions. Our respondents sometimes talked about their sense that some friends rejected them after discovering epilepsy. Just as common, however, were descriptions of good friends treating them no differently because of it. Most thought epilepsy was not important in their established friendships, but that it might tip the balance toward distancing and dissolution with new acquaintances and those thought unable to "handle" such things. The label epilepsy, probably along with most chronic illnesses, was seen as an additional negative feature for those already predisposed to criticize or dislike.

Even for good friends, and sometimes family members, epilepsy and seizures seemed to be difficult topics, to strain interaction, to make it halting, stylized (see Lemert, 1962, on "spurious interaction"), and uncomfortable for all involved. This has been found in previous studies of illness and disability. Fred Davis (1961) studied interaction between physically handicapped people and normals. The latter worked hard *not* to take the handicap into account in the interaction. In a personal account of being physically handicapped, sociologist Irving Zola (1982a) notes similar difficult situations with normals who tried to ignore his leg brace and way of walking. Strauss and Glaser (1975) found that others' knowledge of one's terminal condition made interaction difficult (cf. Comaroff and Maguire, 1981). Myra Bluebond-Langner (1978) devotes much discussion to how children with terminal leukemia, their parents, and hospital staff practiced mutual pretense to keep face-to-face interaction going (see also Glaser and Strauss, 1968). They tacitly agreed that while they all knew the child was dying, no one would act like it. In particular, no one would *talk* about it and other "dangerous topics." In some cases, children themselves would use tactics to keep others away so as to reduce the amount of pretense work that had to be done. This was one way they could exert control over their environment.

Our respondents said that sometimes family and friends found the words "epilepsy" and "seizure" difficult to use. They would ask, obliquely, "Well, how have you been doing?" or "Had any *trouble* lately?", meaning "How is your epilepsy?" or "Have you had any seizures?" Both our respondents and others used many euphemisms for these words. Talking with ill people about their illness may be very hard work for the well.

Respondents' most specific concern about nonfamily relationships focused on employment. The majority believed that if prospective employers discovered their epilepsy and/or seizures, they would not be hired; some thought they might be fired from jobs they held. Work relationships appeared to them to be among the most vulnerable to disclosure of chronic illness.

In some cases, people who had had a seizure at work said that work associates, especially supervisory personnel, never treated them quite the same afterwards. This was less a description of explicit rejection than a withdrawal of trust. It was as though epilepsy and particularly seizures put a person's social competence—one's ability to reciprocate properly in social situations—in doubt. In our respondents' eyes, these others wanted to avoid the chance that they would have to be responsible. Their view was bolstered when they were told they did not meet qualifications for jobs, insurance, driving, and other entitlements because they were too great a risk.

Respondents were also concerned that their seizures might impose on others. While this concern often surfaced in talk about embarrassment and stigma, chronically ill and disabled people may worry that simply *being with* well or able-bodied others is an intrusion. Physically handicapped people may feel this concern when having to ask for help. Our culture makes asking for help not only difficult but also the occasion for incurring debts. The chronically ill and disabled, including our respondents, sense that relationships with friends and associates can be affected by this sense of themselves as a "burden" others must carry. Some manage this by self-imposed isolation, making normalizing relationships all the more difficult to establish.

People with illnesses other than epilepsy experience this same feeling of impaired social competence in others' eyes. Cancer patients and those with multiple sclerosis tell of difficulty in keeping jobs and even friends once their diagnosis is made public (M. Davis, 1973; Winston, 1982). Long-lived national campaigns to "hire the handicapped" attest to the routine discrimination people with physical problems face in getting and keeping employment (see Bogdan and Biklin, 1977). Even sufferers with heart disease express worry over how their employers will receive them after convalescence (e.g. Lear, 1980; Speedling, 1982). Until we know more about how illness figures in these social relationships, our understanding of illness experience will be incomplete.

ILLNESS, SOCIAL MEANINGS,
AND IDENTITY

Illness is a moral experience. When we are sick we soon face new definitions of who we are, what we are capable of, and how others will see us. This is particularly notable for chronic conditions because of their permanence. Sometimes the effects of these definitions are positive. The balance, however, is clearly in the opposite direction.*

Some illnesses, such as epilepsy, are also stigmatized. They carry associated meanings of disgrace and shame beyond the general undesirability of illness itself. Mental illness, leprosy, and venereal disease (lately, herpes) are other examples. Respondents who saw epilepsy as absolutely disgraceful had ready elaborate stories to account for the dread event of a public seizure, for why they took medication, could not drive to some event, and so on. These negative social meanings were often more difficult to contend with than the disease itself (cf. Zola, 1982a; Thomas, 1982).

Confronted by these negative meanings, people tried to shield themselves. Our respondents, and others (see Gussow and Tracey, 1968; Ryan et al., 1980), were often resourceful and successful in concealment and covering strategies. Even those who did not accept negative definitions of themselves often concealed epilepsy for practical reasons, such as getting or keeping a driver's license, job, and insurance.

---

*Some respondents spoke of how having epilepsy made them better people, more sensitive, caring, and understanding of others' problems. The experience of a physical handicap, particularly one that is stable rather than progressive, may provide the person with more of an opportunity to "overcome" than do chronic illnesses defined by downward trajectories or fluctuating uncertainties. In the latter, the biophysiological ground continues to shift, so that one small triumph may be overwhelmed by an even bigger setback in the form of "bad news" from the doctor about a worsened condition (Comaroff and Maguire, 1981).

As with other aspects of illness experience, we have little systematic data on the impact of illness on self and identity. Even when the particular disease is not stigmatized, it can carry with it moral meanings that are consequential (see Waddell, 1982). Susan Sontag (1978) discusses precisely such meanings surrounding tuberculosis in the nineteenth century and cancer today. Irving Zola (1982b) offers a collection of excerpts from first-person accounts of chronic illness and disability experience that give more evidence of this point. Virtually anything that challenges (in others' as well as our own eyes) our capacity or felt capacity to participate in life's worthwhile pursuits is likely to lead to anxieties about our efficacy. Chronic illness and disability are prime examples.

The above discussion is preliminary, a product of what we found in our study of epilepsy together with some considerations raised in other recent studies. With more research on what it is like to be a sick person in society, more systematic and general concepts and connections between ideas will emerge. The appropriate goal would seem to be to accommodate the detail about specific diseases and illnesses, and to reaffirm, expand, and clarify our general understanding of the experience of illness and disability.

SUGGESTIONS FOR CHANGE

We set out in this book to tell the story of what it is like to have epilepsy in our society today. Our strategy, as much as possible, has been to let our respondents' words do that. While we claim no statistical representativeness for our sample, our eighty interviews have allowed us to portray a number of common perceptions, problems, and management strategies that people with epilepsy are likely to experience and pursue.

Our study is intentionally "biased" if by that one means it draws primarily on one point of view (cf. Becker, 1967). We did not aim to portray epilepsy through others' eyes.

Whether that is a liability or an asset depends, to some extent, on the particular audience. Physicians and parents of people with epilepsy, for instance, may find this story does not portray *their* experience of epilepsy at all, or only in a distorted way. If so, we urge them to consider how such different perceptions might come to exist: how, despite perhaps their best efforts to the contrary, some parents and some physicians appear to children and parents more as barriers to successful adaptation than aids or resources. If some parents and physicians do see themselves in these perceptions, we hope they also will ask why.

While in many ways the story of epilepsy may not be a happy one, we believe it is, overall, encouraging. Most of the people we interviewed were not overwhelmed by epilepsy; they did, by and large, cope. Strauss and Glaser's (1975) book on chronic illnesses tells similar stories. Not that this coping was done easily; for many it is always hard work, and there were exceptions. Some people, due to limited material, social, and/or symbolic resources, did not control epilepsy; rather, it seemed to control them. Even those who usually were successful sometimes were not. Almost everyone told of "hard times" with epilepsy; some were experiencing them when we did the interview. Others feared them in the future. Virtually all had struggled to gain some sense of control over epilepsy and its impact on their lives.

We close this story of the experience of epilepsy with some suggestions for how this struggle might be made easier. Although these suggestions are ours, we believe they emerge from our respondents' experience. We intend them as variously provocative ways to put more control of epilepsy and self back in the sufferer's hands. Our suggestions address society, or the public dimension; medical practice, in particular the relationship between the physician and the person with epilepsy; and finally, the individual, or how people with epilepsy themselves manage their illness.

CHANGES IN SOCIETY: THE
PUBLIC IMAGE AND CONTROL
OF EPILEPSY

We asked our respondents what the public image of
epilepsy is. Virtually everyone said it was colored by ignorance and undesirability. A few said others knew that epilepsy is a medical problem and has something to do with
the brain. The public image of epilepsy they saw also reiterated the three myths of heredity (or even contagion!),
psychopathology, and violence discussed in Chapter Two,
and the belief and that people with epilepsy also require
institutionalization.

These diverse themes are all, in one way or another, attached to grand mal seizures. We argued in Chapter Five
that seizures are the signature of epilepsy. We can be more
specific; it is the convulsive, grand mal seizure rather than
other, less dramatic types. People who have epilepsy are
people who have "fits." This image appeared repeatedly in
respondents' comments about others' ideas of epilepsy.
One man said, "I think they get some kind of dreadful disease [image]. This person's going to all of a sudden go into
a fit and go around squeezing someone by the neck or
something." Some believed this grand mal–centered picture of people with epilepsy was perpetuated by mass me-
dia stories connecting it to institutionalization. Another
man said:

> Like I said. I'm 6'10", about 230 pounds. A person
> with epilepsy is supposed to weigh 95 pounds and be
> 5'5" and no muscle, no nothing. That's just the opin-
> ion people have. I don't know if you've ever been to a
> hospital and seen people who really have epilepsy
> bad. They have no control. They are vegetables. They
> cannot do anything. They are the ones you see on
> TV when they talk about epilepsy. No Tom, Dick, or
> Harry who has epilepsy, working in a factory, doing
> fine; like me being a salesman, doing fine. They show

you the ones that's in the hospital, sick. That gives you the image.

A woman described the public image of a person with epilepsy as "someone chained to a wall in the basement . . . somebody that convulses constantly."

Sociologist Patrick West (1982) suggests this idea that epilepsy *is* grand mal seizures should be a target of educational efforts by physicians and self-help groups. One way to combat this narrow and extreme definition is to make it clear that seizures happen to people who do not have epilepsy, and that epilepsy includes many different types of seizures/symptoms, not just the grand mal type.

While the public image of epilepsy has improved, much work remains to be done. There should be concerted attempts to normalize and diversify the public picture of epilepsy. Public education and public service announcements about epilepsy are a step in the right direction. The Epilepsy Foundation of America and other groups have fielded televised announcements, showing public personalities giving information about epilepsy or even identifying themselves as having it. These efforts are quite recent. Startlingly few of our respondents could name anybody "famous" who has or has had epilepsy, or could recall seeing such announcements. Perhaps first-aid techniques for someone having a seizure could be taught and disseminated through campaigns similar to those for cardiopulmonary resuscitation (CPR) or the now-common Heimlich maneuver.

There is some controversy, however, about using chronically ill and/or disabled "stars" as ways to communicate information to the public about a disease or disability. These people are portrayed as winners, as victors in a battle against the condition. The problem, as Zola (1982a) has noted, is that most people with these illnesses and disabilities are not accurately described as "victorious," but rather as coping with, but sometimes being overwhelmed by, their problems. The stars who speak for the thousands who are never seen have themselves become (honorary) normals; they have overcome. This definition actually contradicts the meaning of chronic, and distorts the actual experience of illness lived "behind the scenes." We need more images of regular people leading lives in spite of or with their conditions, as the man above says, "working in the factory, doing fine; like me being a salesman, doing fine."

While we may dispute the means of educating, simply conveying the word "epilepsy" to public audiences may be progress. The goal should be to present truthful information and images about epilepsy and the people who have it—to show the diversity behind the label, and not to deny the word. Medical euphemisms, such as "convulsive disorder," may produce an effect precisely the opposite of that intended. To cover something up is to admit it brings disgrace. Epilepsy should be a word, as one woman put it, that is part of "kitchen, every day conversation. Not some grandiose medical thing." Finally, the audiences for these messages should contain the significant number of people who themselves suffer in secrecy with epilepsy. It is not only naïve others who must be educated; it is often the afflicted themselves.

A second and related area for change is the systematic and sometimes official discrimination. These disenfranchisements in employment, insurance, and driving shore up the stereotypes and prejudicial thinking described in this book. They are part of the devalued moral status of epilepsy. They become (independent of what people actually *can* do) evidence of its disabling impact. People with epilepsy *must* be dangerous, out of control, if they cannot get a driver's license or "work around machines," or if they are such risks that insurance companies will not issue them financial protection. Like deviants who suffer general rather than limited disreputability in the public eye, people with epilepsy have faced, and continue to face, categoric ineligibility for certain jobs, prerogatives, and protections.

While these questions of eligibility may be complex in

some cases, such categoric disenfranchisements bring undue hardship. There is much room for improved public regulation and control. Official and private (but pervasive) rules and regulations regarding epilepsy must strike a considerably more equitable balance between the interests of individuals and those of the state and/or other organizations. Only when a job requires skills and competencies *the person under review* can be shown not to possess should *that person* be held ineligible for *that job*. Only when *this person's* seizures make driving demonstrably unsafe should he or she be refused a license. Moreover, just as we now have specific restrictions on license holders requiring eye glasses, for example, people who have seizures only during their sleep could have licenses restricted to daytime driving.* Only when specific features of a person's medical biography (not merely the diagnosis alone) can be shown to increase significantly chances of accident or injury should *that person* be a problem for insurers.

This view flies in the face of the usual ways we award eligibility and entitlement. Laws and policies are supposed to apply to categories of people in universalistic and impartial ways (quite aside from what actually happens). These practices are assumed to insure equity and fairness. We think it as likely that they bring just the opposite, namely, injustice and despair at being treated capriciously and arbitrarily. It is only when we begin to appreciate the human impact of bureaucratic, "impersonal" policies, as well as how they support more diffuse social devaluation of people with epilepsy, that we will be stirred to change.

---

*There are no systematic data to show that epilepsy causes increased automobile accidents. There have been some promising developments recently around driver's licensing. Some states have removed the blanket and arbitrary requirements about being seizure-free for a specific period. Instead, people must present medical certification that they are able to drive without undue risk. The effects of these changed laws should be monitored (they do make the physician even more responsible).

CHANGES IN MEDICAL PRACTICE: DOCTORS AND PATIENTS AS PARTNERS

The most common, typical thing doctors do for people with epilepsy is to prescribe and monitor medications to stabilize or reduce their seizures. They of course do other things too, but this is the center of routine medical treatment for epilepsy. Patients are supposed to do what doctors say, reaping the benefits of improved condition and lessened auxiliary problems. This is the prevailing wisdom surrounding not just the medical care of people with epilepsy, but medical care in general. Doctors direct; patients follow; improved health and stability result.

Aside from often being simply wrong, this doctor-centered view of medical practice assumes that the most important thing, perhaps the *only* thing, patients must do is to listen carefully to and follow their doctors' orders. A sizeable literature on the importance of social and social psychological factors in illness to the contrary, this view continues to predominate. It may be in part *because of* this literature on the social "factors," "aspects," and "variables" in illness that this wisdom persists, not only in the world of medicine, but in the larger culture. Seeing the significance of social phenomena in illness in terms of "factors," "aspects," and "variables" misses precisely the point we have been making in this book. Illness is not something in which there are "social factors"; it is itself *profoundly social* as a phenomenon for study. These diluted and vague substitutes for "cause" reflect common social epidemiological thinking. Accordingly, "social factors" in illness are those conditions external to the body and mind that influence the incidence and course of *disease*. This is fundamentally a medically-oriented perspective. It is much too narrow to allow us to appreciate illness as we have discussed it.

Physicians need at least to consider that illness often may be only loosely linked to disease, and that it is at least as complex as the disease itself. While physicians are experts in the treatment of disease and disorder, can they claim to "treat" the social experience of illness? What would such treatment be? How, for instance, could a doctor "treat" the relationships of dependence that developed with family members, or the way others respond to witnessing a seizure, or the person's perception of the stigma surrounding epilepsy? How would such treatment accommodate the new insights into suffering some said they had developed? Indeed, how could a medical doctor expect, or be expected, to minister to the diverse and sometimes contradictory feelings and needs not only of the patient, but of all those others who make up the experience of illness? The answer is clear: for the most part he or she cannot.

This view has implications for the medical treatment of epilepsy. Most respondents told us that their experience with doctors was one-sided; routine visits include a brief physical examination, a series of familiar questions (few answers), and a reissue or alteration of prescriptions. This is medical treatment for the disorder (disease) epilepsy. But these people were also "ill." Respondents felt doctors often were "just going through the motions" without really attending to or even hearing their problems and concerns. These physicians, had they had a chance to speak for themselves, undoubtedly would see it differently. What can be done about this apparent impasse or unconnectedness between people with epilepsy and their doctors?

We believe doctors and patients with epilepsy need to be coparticipants in treatment rather than continuing the disease-expert-and-disordered-body approach typical of this care. People with epilepsy must pursue this participation and shared responsibility for their own care. We found evidence that most of our respondents were trying to do just that. It seems likely, however, that a large part of the initiative for more systematic coparticipation must come from the doctor.

Doctors must acknowledge that illness is something too complex for any single person, no matter how highly trained, to manage. They should be expert at what they are trained to do—to control disease—but they should also encourage patients, and others willing and able to contribute, to share the responsibility of managing illness. This entails listening carefully to their patients' concerns about seizures, self, the future, the meanings of medications, stigma, relationships of dependence and, perhaps most difficult, about relationships with the doctors themselves. In short, doctors must not only ask questions and give directions, they must give answers and take directions as members of a collectivity, all of whom are responsible for managing illness.

CHANGES IN THE LIFE: OWNING EPILEPSY AND REALIZING SELF

A brighter future for people with epilepsy depends on their gaining ownership and control over their illness. This means first and foremost that they acknowledge their epilepsy as part of them and, having done so, deny it to others as grounds for devaluing definitions and treatment. This must be done *by* people with epilepsy *for* themselves *without* significant reliance on outsiders, most particularly professionals. As long as people who have epilepsy see it as shameful or as something to be hidden (for whatever reason) *and then proceed to hide it*, they will be captive to it. The "it" here is the complex of social meanings attached to the medical diagnosis, what we called in Chapter Two the "historical and social realities of epilepsy." There are several elements to such a bold step forward. We suggest those most apparent to us. There are undoubtedly others.

People with epilepsy (indeed, all persons with chronic illness) must put more trust in their own capacities to know and understand their bodies and body-related feelings. It is possible that our highly technologized society actually discourages us from believing in our own experience as a guide to judgments about how to live our lives and care for ourselves. Our data show that people do develop and use this knowledge (often unsystematically and uncritically) even though they may not see what they do as ethno or lay medicine. We believe this offers promising possibilities, nonetheless.

An available model for the development and use of lay medical knowledge is the women's self-help movement, incorporating particular knowledge about and care of reproductive processes and birthing (see Boston Women's Health Book Collective, 1973; Ruzek, 1979). The history of this movement is filled with conflict, despair, and triumph for women who view their struggle in terms of regaining control of their "bodies and selves" from a variety of service professionals and institutions, primarily, doctors and hospitals (see also Wertz and Wertz, 1977). For people with epilepsy, the single most important lesson here is the very success of women's self help. Competent, efficient, and safe lay care *can* exist.

There are other examples of successful political movements that people with epilepsy might consider. One that is congenial because it turns on limitations of the body is the "independent living movement" by and for people with physical handicaps, including people otherwise considered totally debilitated (see DeJong, 1979; Zola, 1979). More distant in substance but not in theme and purpose are the black civil rights movement of the 1960s, the women's movement, gay liberation, and even the Gray Panthers. These movements suggest that people with ostensibly devalued characteristics can themselves effect dramatic improvements in how they are defined and treated, if not in widespread and immediate popular support, then in terms of new or enforced rights legislation. The past two decades have witnessed many such groups effectively opposing and rejecting conventional negative definitions (see Kitsuse,

1980; Anspach, 1979). Social separation and isolation of illness makes the development of such movements difficult but not impossible.

One barrier to similar success for people with epilepsy is the absence of a subculture similar to those that nurtured these movements. People with epilepsy are isolated in their own private closets. Most of the people we interviewed said they did not even know another person with the disorder. Only a handful had been to a meeting of a local chapter of one of the national voluntary associations for epilepsy. The ideology of self help, so central to the success of the women's health movement, was virtually absent, although there is growing interest and participation in epilepsy self-help organizations in the United States (see Borman et al., 1980; Self-Help Development Institute, 1980). Before people with epilepsy individually and collectively can hope to own and manage their condition they must begin to find one another. This means talking about epilepsy.

We are not suggesting, naïvely, wholesale and unselective disclosure. Unfortunately, official and unofficial discrimination is still very much a part of our society. The stigma associated with epilepsy is not only a historical but also a contemporary reality (although this stigma apparently has lessened with time). We feel confident, however, that in order to get beyond epilepsy people must externalize it in talk to others, at first carefully chosen; later, we hope, such careful choice will be unnecessary. Respondents who recalled the experience of telling someone close to them about their epilepsy assure us of the soundness of this recommendation.

Talking about epilepsy is externalizing it. Externalizing it is sharing it. Worrisome things about us that we and others can together carry become less a burden and more a mere facet of our selves—one among a number of things about us. We speak of "getting it off my chest" or apologizing to others for "dumping all this" on them. Such phrases are telling. People who told others about their epilepsy felt decidedly better because of it; telling was therapeutic. The longer concealment lasts and the more complicated it becomes, the heavier the weight, the greater the significance of epilepsy in one's life. Those who seemed to manage their epilepsy to their greatest advantage were those who had *defined* it as of minimal importance to them. Virtually all of them talked with at least some others regularly about it. Epilepsy, like sex and death, must be made speakable not just behind closed doors among a select few, but at all levels of society. It is only then that we can begin to banish the ghosts that have for so long made it so mysterious and threatening.

Appendix

DOING THE STUDY: ISSUES, PROBLEMS, AND STRATEGIES

This study was conceived out of our interest in the relationship between deviance and illness. For several years we were immersed in a research project examining the historical origins and consequences of the medicalization of deviance (Conrad and Schneider, 1980). During this period we had long discussions about the connections between illness and deviance, mostly from the perspective of medicalizing deviance. We began to see that if we wanted to understand the relationship of deviance and illness, we would need to analyze the problem from both sides. We had investigated many examples of medicalized deviance, but what would be its opposite? It became clear that what we were seeking was a conception of deviant or stigmatized illness (Gussow and Tracey, 1968): an illness in which the sufferers were treated *as if* they were deviant. A few examples came to mind, including leprosy, venereal disease, and epilepsy. Because of its history as a stigmatized problem and its prevalence, we settled on epilepsy as our subject for research. In the beginning, our interest in epilepsy came mainly from our theoretical interests.

In collaboration with a third colleague, Rita Dohrmann, who herself had epilepsy, we began meeting regularly to decide how to proceed in our research. At first, our goals were modest: ten or fifteen interviews simply to get some sense of how people managed epilepsy and stigma. But before long, our study was transformed into something much more. The data from our first dozen or so interviews were so fascinating that we put our original theoretical interests on a back burner and focused our research directly on exploring the experience of epilepsy. Our third colleague left the project to pursue other interests, while we plodded on for several years collecting and analyzing data. This appendix discusses some of the major issues and problems of the research. We hope it serves as both a research retrospective and a guide for others.

STUDYING THE EXPERIENCE OF ILLNESS

We can summarize our approach to studying illness experience as follows: 1) collect data systematically; 2) develop a nonclinic sample; 3) present a sociologically-rendered, "insider's" view of the experience, and 4) be both specific and analytic.

To collect data systematically we developed an interview guide and then set out to locate an appropriate sample. Throughout the first twenty interviews we revised the guide several times as we added or deleted items depending on what we learned from each interview and how effectively they produced rich and detailed information. The final version consisted of fifty open-ended questions. It can be found at the end of this Appendix. Our goal was to elicit clear and detailed responses. In consequence, we were somewhat flexible in creating and using the interview guide. For instance, in any interview we covered all the items, but not necessarily in the order presented. Our goal was to make data collection more a guided conversation than a survey. Tape recording the interviews and then having them typed (the major research expense, aside from our own time) insured accuracy and completeness of the data.

Because our main interest was how people experience and manage epilepsy, we wanted to interview people outside hospital and medical settings. Except for some seizure-related injuries and initial diagnosis and/or medication monitoring none of our respondents had been institutionalized for epilepsy. We attempted to include a broad range of people and life experiences. By interviewing most people at home, we could underscore that ours was a non-medical study and about epilepsy in their everyday lives.

To the degree possible, we wanted to present an insider's view of illness experience, as it is lived by the ill. Broadly speaking, our research was influenced by the symbolic interactionist and phenomenological traditions in that we emphasize the importance of meaning and first-hand accounts in understanding social life.

Finally, we wanted our research to contribute to knowledge in two ways. First, we wanted to remain true to the subject of study and thus present a detailed description of what it is like to have epilepsy. Second, we wanted to extend the sociological understanding of illness experience. This goal led us to look for conceptual understanding in the specific epilepsy data that would suggest connections to other kinds of illness experience.

In the following sections we elaborate some of the issues that arose and strategies we used regarding sampling, interviewing, and the analysis and writing in this project.

WHO TO STUDY: SAMPLING

Deciding who to study seemed straightforward, but actually accomplishing this involved a variety of conceptual as well as practical considerations. Do we interview people who are already diagnosed as having epilepsy? Does this mean we accept the medical definition of the disorder, neglecting those interesting and important people who may have a condition that could be diagnosed as epilepsy but who have never sought medical treatment? Following Howard Becker (1973), we might call these people "potential epileptics." The Commission Report (1978) suggests that up to 25 percent of all people with epilepsy do not receive medical treatment. A recent epidemiological study of prisoners (Whitman et al., 1982) found a prevalence rate of 2.4 percent, significantly higher than that reported in the epilepsy literature. Although these "potential epileptics" are surely sociologically interesting, our concern with the experience of *having epilepsy* directed us to focus on people who at sometime had been diagnosed as having the condition or who believed they had it.

As it turned out, all our respondents received a diagnosis of epilepsy or "convulsive disorder" at some point in their lives, and roughly 90 percent were still taking seizure control medication. Since we made no checks on our respondents' medical records, it is possible that people could fabricate a history of epilepsy. Given the breadth and depth of our interviews, however, we think such an account would be easily detectable. Even if one or two respondents said they had epilepsy who a neurologist would not so diagnose, they still experienced the social and personal consequences of having epilepsy if they and others defined them to have it.

Locating and constructing a sample was not an easy task. Our first six respondents were referred to us by a local self-help group. We wanted to expand beyond this unrepresentative group (few people with epilepsy join self-help groups), so we placed classified advertisements in local and university newspapers, and shoppers. The ad read: "EPILEPSY. Drake University sociologists studying people's experiences with epilepsy. Need volunteers to interview. Confidentiality assured. Call . . ." The shoppers' papers brought the largest response, from both women and men. We attempted to enlarge our sample by asking each respondent to pass on a letter about the study with a returnable postcard to any person with epilepsy that they knew (a copy of this letter is at the end of this Appendix). Very few people knew others with epilepsy, although we did obtain a few respondents this way. To tap another population, we asked a local vocational rehabilitation agency to solicit clients with epilepsy who would be willing to be interviewed. We received ten respondents in this manner.

Several times during the research we approached neurologists about our study. The three neurologists with whom we discussed our research were enthusiastic and promised either to give their patients letters of introduction about the study or refer to us names of patients willing to be interviewed. Despite all the enthusiasm, we did not obtain a single respondent through physicians. Perhaps clinical care and busy practices prevailed, precluding attention to the research interests of two sociologists.

Our sample is of course limited by its self-selected nature. We interviewed people who answered our ads or who were willing to speak with us. Even if we wanted a random sample, no available lists of people with epilepsy exist from which to draw one. We attempted to develop as broadly based a sample as we could. We not only used sex, age, and occupation as measures of our breadth, but also sampled theoretically as the interviewing progressed. We tried to interview people from a variety of socioeconomic

backgrounds and occupations, and with diverse experience with medical services. To the extent possible we
sampled experiences, events, and perceptions more than
persons with this or that characteristic.

Our final sample of eighty people (forty-four women
and thirty-six men) includes a cross section of those with
epilepsy. Our respondents tended to be young (average
age twenty-eight) and middle to lower-middle class in
terms of income (43 percent earning less than $11,000;
36 percent between $11,000 and $22,000). The distribution in terms of education is somewhat more "middle":
only 5 percent had not completed high school, 26 percent
had completed a trade or vocational school; 32 percent
had taken some college work, 25 percent had completed
college; 8 percent had completed graduate or professional
education. Most of our respondents were either working
or going to school at the time of the interview, but eleven
people (14 percent) said they currently were unemployed
and looking for work.

Most said they had had grand mal seizures.* Some of
our respondents said they had not had a seizure in several
years; others reported them as weekly events. Several had
been diagnosed virtually at birth, others in middle age.
Twenty-five percent said their diagnosis came before adolescence; 44 percent were diagnosed during adolescence;
7 percent were diagnosed while young adults, and 15 percent as adults. Collectively, our respondents had had a
good deal of experience with epilepsy, specifically, over
1,000 years all together. The average duration of this experience was thirteen years. A few said they had been diagnosed within weeks of the interview; one man had had epilepsy for thirty-seven years.

---

*We did not sample by type of seizure, although all types appeared
to be represented. One of the most significant aspects of seizures, as it
turned out, was not the frequency but rather when they occurred. People with solely nocturnal seizures had considerably less management
problems than others did.

At one point we wanted to extend the age range of our sample by interviewing some elderly people. After calling a dozen nursing homes it became apparent that elderly people with epilepsy whom we could interview would be difficult to find. None had answered our ads. Several nursing homes said they either could not give permission for us to interview their patients, or that the patients were not coherent enough to be interviewed. The calls to nursing homes yielded one prospective respondent, and as our research drew to a close we abandoned the search for elderly respondents.

One unexpected discovery was that for at least six respondents we were the first people other than their doctor and immediate family members with whom they talked about epilepsy. For another half dozen we were among the very few with whom they ever had discussed it. These people with such secretive strategies added an important dimension to the study and broadened our understanding of both epilepsy and illness. We believe people do not readily discuss their illnesses with others in their everyday lives. For most of our respondents, our interview was the most prolonged discussion about epilepsy they had ever had. They said they appreciated the opportunity to talk freely to an interested person about their disorder. We feel our respondents were quite open and frank about their feelings and perceptions.

We did not begin the research with a predetermined number of interviews in mind. When we applied for funding we suggested a goal of one hundred, but after sixty interviews, it became clear that we were hearing many similar stories. The last twenty interviews were given to two sampling tasks: including more men to more equalize the sample's sex distribution and interviewing people in another part of the country to see if there were any regional or cultural differences apparent in respondents' experiences.

Our eighty interviews yielded over 2,000 pages of single-spaced transcripts—a virtual mountain of data to

read, code, and analyze. In retrospect, fifty interviews probably would have been sufficient, although some of our
most interesting and stimulating respondents were among
the last thirty people interviewed. While nearly all our respondents added something to our understanding of epilepsy, nine or ten particularly articulate people contributed decidedly to our insights. Locating these respondents
was a combination of luck, self-selection, and a sufficient
number of interviews.

HOW TO COLLECT DATA:
INTERVIEWING

We interviewed about 80 percent of our respondents
in their homes (the remainder in our offices). Typically the
interviews took place in the respondents' living rooms or
at a kitchen table over coffee or tea. We guided the interview, asking questions, probing responses, and comment-
ing to encourage people to tell their stories. Usually our
interviews followed our guide's format, going from general
to specific questions and covering a variety of topics concerning epilepsy. We tried, as much as possible, to make
the interview a relaxed, comfortable conversation.

We tape recorded all the interviews. This allowed us to
maintain eye contact, which encouraged easy and detailed
conversation, and also saved us from writer's cramp. When
a research topic is as broad as ours was, we encourage using a tape recorder. Brief periods of intense and highly important conversation are full of complex meaning that is
easily missed when having to record talk manually. Equally
important, taping insured greater accuracy in capturing
our respondents' words. In virtually no case was the small
cassette recorder a hindrance; everyone seemed not to notice it once the interview began. Three people, however,
gave us added information only after the recorder was
turned off. Several commented that they were glad we
were taping because they did not want to be misquoted.

A few words should be said about the data our interviews produced. Research of this type relies heavily on what people say, to the neglect of what they actually do (see Deutscher, 1973). Although we checked our interviews for internal consistency, by and large we took people at their word (as do most interviewers). Because our questions asked about events and experiences that may have occurred several years before, it is likely that a certain amount of retrospective interpretation, as well as simple forgetting, colored what people said. Respondents often interpret past events from the present context and then report them in this light. Even given the limits of such data, the open-ended interview is the most appropriate and efficient way to talk to a large number of people about their experience of illness. Because our emphasis was on *experience*, the problem of words versus deeds and of retrospective interpretation are of little significance. We wanted people's current perceptions of their lives and situations.

We should also mention that we overlooked an important area of life in constituting and constructing the interview guide. Only after we completed our interviews did we realize that we omitted specific questions about sexuality. A few respondents mentioned it in other contexts, but as Zola's (1982a) book poignantly shows, sexuality can be a significant aspect of illness experience.

MAKING SENSE OF THE DATA: ANALYSIS

In this type of research it is ideal to do coding and analysis as the data are collected. Because we both were involved in another project, along with routine but substantial teaching obligations, this was impossible to do. In an attempt to compensate, we from the first listened to each other's interviews and edited the transcripts for accuracy as well as for insight. In addition, we wrote theoretical memoranda (Glaser, 1978) throughout, developing links between substantive detail and what we thought was going on, sociologically, in these descriptions. These memos proved invaluable when we started the final coding and analysis.

We began coding the interviews by reading carefully a sample of the transcripts to develop both substantive and general topic codes. These included such codes as diagnosis, prediagnosis, discovery, doctors, medication, family, dependence, driving, control, seizures, stigma, concealing, and others' ideas about epilepsy. We then photocopied the original transcripts, marked each appropriate line or section with the code in the margin, and cut up and filed the pieces of paper according to the codes. Within each of the more general categories was a number of subcategories which we marked on each excerpt with different colored pencils. These subcategories were more thematic than substantive; for example, for the doctors' chapter the coding included the following:

1. Organization and diagnosis
   a. First visit; hospital
2. Information exchange
   a. Ambivalence and feelings toward doctors
3. Medical versus social problems
   a. Scariness
4. When would you consult a doctor?
5. Others

The coding and analysis took a great deal of time—two full summers, plus any time we could set aside during the school year.

Fairly early in our project it became apparent that the medical perspective on epilepsy did very little to describe our respondents' experience. Our data indicated clearly that a sociological analysis based on epilepsy experience would highlight a different reality of epilepsy than does the dominant medical definition. Based on our early findings, we wrote a paper that set out how such an approach to epilepsy might look (Schneider and Conrad, 1981). As analysis was under way, we wrote another paper focusing specifically on how people with epilepsy manage stigma (Schneider and Conrad, 1980). The latter paper is absorbed in this book (Chapter Seven), while the former remains independent of this book, although closely related.

Although we looked for themes and common experiences, it is important to value the uniqueness of each person's story. We did not exclude a respondent's story on the grounds that it was unique; indeed, the unique experience could give voice to a more common one. For example, the woman who did not tell her husband about epilepsy even though they had been married seventeen years provided perspective for less extreme concealing strategies. The woman who said she learned how to manage her epilepsy from the example of her diabetic husband, who switched urine with a friend before a job screening exam, made us see the existence and at least one function of an illness "underground."

Selecting the quotes for this book was a difficult task. The quotes are critical to making the analytic themes of the book grounded and clear but there were no simple formulas for selecting and using them. As it evolved, our research began and ended with the quotes, first as a source of themes and then as a pool of specific illustrations for them. We chose our illustrative quotes on the basis of their clarity, richness of descriptive material, and resonance with the point being made. Often one quote can represent the experience of many persons; at other times it seems important to present the individual variation or "deviant case" to show how exceptions actually often support the pattern.

We used more than 350 excerpted quotes in this book. Words from nearly all of our respondents can be found someplace in the book. After we completed the manuscript we tallied the distribution of quotes over all eighty interviews. Seventy-three of our eighty respondents were quoted at least once, thirty-eight at least four times, and ten were quoted eight or more times. The most frequently-cited respondent was quoted in seventeen places. These counts show that the data used are distributed widely over our sample of respondents.

Collaborating in research and writing has both rewards and frustrations. Certainly, a shared intellectual perspective on what is being done, how, and why it is important is essential. Such consensus, however, even among those who work closely together, cannot be assumed. It must be negotiated throughout the work. We discussed all important issues about analysis and coding, themes of this paper or that chapter, how one part of the book fit or did not fit with another, and so on. We continued the practice we had developed in our earlier joint work of writing chapters separately, then criticizing and editing one another's writing.

ROADS NOT TAKEN

The strategy we chose for investigating the experience of illness is not the only one possible for such research. Had we been able to use other strategies as well, our research undoubtedly would have been enriched. Given our limited resources, however, using these strategies would have required a much smaller and narrower sample.

We interviewed each of our respondents only once. Interviewing each person a second or third time (say six months and a year later) would have added a longitudinal dimension to our study and allowed us to examine how illness experience changed over time. Fred Davis (1963) used this strategy in his study of polio victims. Another variation would have been to create a few detailed life histories, based on perhaps ten or fifteen hours of interviews with the same people, to portray the experience more in terms of biography (for example, Bogdan and Taylor, 1982). Such case studies increase specificity and depth, but risk being atypical and idiosyncratic. Our goal of a broadly-based and systematic investigation, coupled with the limited time and material resources, made developing such life histories impossible.

We only present the sufferer's perspective of illness experience. By interviewing family members and others we could have explored more how the family influenced illness experience and how the illness and sick person affected the family. Speedling's (1982) study of heart attack victims, for instance, examines such questions.

Participant-observation research presents some possibilities for studying the experience of illness, although it has been used rarely in noninstitutional settings. This may be due in part to the absence of any "illness subcultures" and to the scarcity of "illness communities" available for convenient study. One strategy might be to begin with participant observation in a clinical setting and then to follow the patients into the community with regular visits and interviews (see Speedling, 1982). Self-help groups are another potential site for participant observation. One of our graduate students conducted a small research project in epilepsy self-help groups (Pillemer, 1981), but these groups remain special and limited samples of people with epilepsy. Perhaps the most difficult and challenging strategy would be to study people in their everyday lives. This means doing observation at home and work, and following people over a period of time in their daily rounds. Such a sample, both in the number of respondents and in the segment of life observed, would be small, but the distinct advantage would be a direct view of people's lives in natural settings. Jules Henry's (1971) study of families with emotionally disturbed children is provocative in this regard. Ideally, some combination of systematic depth interviewing, life histories, and participant observation would enable researchers to examine in depth still unexplored regions of illness experience.

INTERVIEW GUIDE

I would like to ask you some questions about having epilepsy. I would appreciate answers as full, complete and detailed as possible. There is no need to rush, so we can discuss any of the questions or topics at length. In our attempt to be comprehensive in gathering information, some of the questions may overlap in the information they seek. If you find this to be the case, please bear with me. If you have any questions during the interview, please feel free to ask them. The following questions serve mainly as a guide and you should not feel limited by them in any way.

1. How did you first discover you had epilepsy? [Probe: seizure, medical identification, etc.; when? where?]

2. Tell me how you felt when you found out you had epilepsy. What did you do?

3. Before this first realization that you had epilepsy, did you ever suspect you might have this disorder? Tell me about that. [Probe: How so, what cues? What did you do about it?]

4. When were you medically diagnosed and by whom? What led you to go to a physician in the first place? Do you have any other medical problems or difficulties in addition to your epilepsy? [Probe: chronic, psychiatric, etc.]

5. Before you were medically diagnosed, did anyone ever suggest to you that you might have epilepsy or might get epilepsy? [If yes] What were the circumstances? What was said and what was the response?

6. Did you ever have seizures *before* you were medically diagnosed? [If yes] Tell me about it. What did you think was going on? How did you handle the situation?

7. Have you ever been hospitalized—been in the hospital at least overnight—because of your epilepsy? Tell me about that. [Probe: When, where, what were the circumstances?] [If no] What happened when you had seizures?

8. Tell me about the doctor who told you you had epilepsy. [Pause for response] How did he or she decide that

you had epilepsy? Do you remember what the doctor told you about it?

9. Do you see a doctor regularly for your epilepsy? How often? Tell me about going to see the doctor—what does he or she do, say; how does the doctor act? [If no] Did you sometime in the past see a doctor regularly? When was that? How did you happen to see him or her in the first place?

10. [If person does see a doctor or "has" a doctor] How do you feel about your doctor and his or her relationship with you now?

11. How do you feel physicians in general have treated you and your epilepsy?

12. Under what circumstances or conditions would you contact a physician for your epilepsy now?

13. Are you currently taking any medicine for your epilepsy? [If no] Have you ever in the past taken medicine for your epilepsy? [If no, skip to question 18]

14. Do you know what the medicine is that you are taking or have taken for your epilepsy? How often do you take it? (or, did you take it?) Do you take it regularly?

15. Did you ever miss taking your medicine? [Clarify—I mean not take it because you forgot or couldn't or something else] What happened? [Probe]

16. How do you feel about having to take this medicine for your epilepsy? What do you think that this medicine does for you? What happens to you, how do you feel when you take this medicine? What effects does it have on you? [Probe: Any "side effects" or effects in addition to the apparent control of seizures?]

17. Have you ever considered not taking your medicine or stopping your visits to the doctor? [Probe: I mean on purpose, intentionally. Tell me about it.]

18. Did discovering you have epilepsy affect your life? Try to describe how it has, or, if it has not, why it hasn't. [Probe: Think about how your life was before you found out you had epilepsy.]

19. When you discovered you had epilepsy, were there any changes you had to make in your life? Tell me about them. [If yes] Why did you have to make these changes? [Probe: Seek whether these changes are due to family, friends, job, school, marriage, having children, etc., or relating to them.]

20. At first, when you found out you had epilepsy, did you talk with your family, friends, employer (teacher) and others about it? Who did you talk to and what did you tell them? How did they respond? [Probe]

21. Do you talk with people now—particularly new people you meet—about your epilepsy? What do you say and how do they react?

22. How do other people, if they do, become aware that you have epilepsy? Do you tell them?

23. Under what conditions or in what kinds of situations do you tell other people about your epilepsy? In what situations do you *not* talk about it with others?

24. Does it matter to you that other people know you have epilepsy? Tell me about it.

25. Do you think that people relate to you differently after they find out (or know) you have epilepsy? [Clarify "people"—all, some, who? Also ask how they do relate differently, if so.] Do *you* relate or act differently around people who know you have epilepsy?

26. Have you ever concealed the fact that you have epilepsy in a situation where information is requested or expected about it? [If yes, ask for description of situations and how they were handled; if no, ask specifically about driver's license, job, school, etc.]

27. Do you think that people can tell by looking at you or being around you that you have epilepsy? How do you think they know? What do you do about it?

28. Tell me about seizures. What are they? What happens to you? How do you know? How do you feel about seizures?

29. Has a seizure ever caused you problems in social

situations? [Probe: In public? At work? Where?] With what people and what kinds of problems?

30. Does having a seizure in the presence of others affect their behavior toward you? In what ways, both immediately and in terms of their future interaction with you?

31. Do you know when a seizure is coming? How? What do you do in such situations? [Probe: Ask for a description.]

32. Does it matter that you don't know much ahead of time when a seizure is about to occur? Tell me, how do you deal with that? What do you do?

33. Are there situations when you think a seizure is more likely to occur? Tell me about these situations, what are they like? [Probe: Ask for description.] How do you handle these situations? Do you try to avoid them? What do you do if you can't avoid them? [Probe: Look for strategies in such situations.]

34. How long has it been since your last seizure? How often do you have seizures? Do you know what kind of seizures you have? Where did you find out?

35. Your last seizure was ———. [If long ago] That was some time ago. Do you still think you have epilepsy? Why?

36. Do you carry anything with you that could identify you as having epilepsy? Like a bracelet, a card, tongue depressor?

37. Have you ever seen someone have a seizure? [If yes] Please describe it and how you felt and responded.

38. Overall, how has epilepsy affected your life? [Probe: What kind of difficulties it caused in life, family, friends, work.] Has having epilepsy ever kept you from doing anything you wanted to do? Tell me about that. [Probe also regarding school, marriage plans]

39. Are there, or have there been, any periods or situations in your life when having epilepsy has been especially difficult or troublesome? Tell me about them, please.

40. Has having epilepsy affected your choice of a job or career? How so?

41. Do you know any other persons with epilepsy? Have you discussed epilepsy with them? What types of things did you discuss? Are these persons your friends, family members; who are they?

42. Have you ever considered seeking professional services—other than from your doctor—or information about epilepsy, or joining a group of other people with epilepsy or seeking information from such a group? Why or why not?

43. Can you think of any advantages you have experienced from having epilepsy? Tell me about them.

44. Do you think there are any differences between the ideas of "being an epileptic" and "having epilepsy"? Do you think of yourself as an epileptic?

45. Have your family members, close friends, or employers made any adjustments in their lives or situations to help you to cope with having epilepsy? [If yes] What are they—what kinds of things have they done?

46. Have any of these people done things, unintentionally, to make having epilepsy difficult for you? Tell me about these things.

47. Do you think anyone has done anything *intentionally* to make it more difficult for you to cope with having epilepsy? [If yes] Who are these people and what kinds of things have they done?

48. In general, what do you think other people, people who do not have epilepsy, think about it? Do you think they know what epilepsy is?

49. Can you think of any famous individuals or public figures who had or have epilepsy?

50. Is there anything else that you would like to tell me about what it is like to have epilepsy?

LETTER PASSED TO ANONYMOUS PEOPLE WITH EPILEPSY

Dear Person:

Recently an acquaintance of yours told us that he or she knew someone who had been medically diagnosed as having epilepsy. This person did not tell us your name or anything about you and we have no way of identifying you. We would, however, like to ask you to help us in a study we are doing of the life experiences of people with epilepsy.

We are two sociologists from Drake University and have no connections to state or local agencies or medical personnel whatsoever. We appreciate the fact that you might be somewhat reticent about identifying yourself publicly as having epilepsy. We are interested in studying and learning more about the reasons why and the ways in which people who have epilepsy sometimes face discrimination and prejudiced attitudes. We would like to interview you (confidentially, of course) to learn more about the social and personal experiences, perceptions, problems and adjustments people who have epilepsy face in our society. We think the results of our research will be helpful to others who have epilepsy as well as those who do not. Our research is partly funded by the Epilepsy Foundation of America and a subdivision of the Department of Health, Education, and Welfare.

If you would agree to be interviewed by one of us, all of the information we collect would be held in the strictest of confidence. All such material would be coded numerically and access to this information would be allowed only to the two persons conducting this research.

If you would agree to be interviewed, we could arrange to meet any place of your choice that is reasonably quiet where we could stay for about an hour. Our offices here at Drake are always available for such interviews. To assure accuracy and completeness, we would record the interview and then transcribe these recordings into type-written form. We would appreciate very much your help in this project.

If you agree to be interviewed, please write your first name and telephone number on the enclosed postcard and return it to us. We will then call you and set up a date and time for the interview. If you have some questions you would like to ask before agreeing to be interviewed, please call Joseph Schneider at ————.

Again, we don't know who you are. We have sent this letter and its envelope to the person who knows you and he or she has forwarded it. Thank you for your consideration and we hope to be hearing from you.

Sincerely,

Joseph W. Schneider, Ph.D.   Peter Conrad, Ph.D.

References

Alonzo, Angelo.   1979.   "Everyday illness behavior: A situational approach to health status deviations."   *Social Science and Medicine* 13A:397–404.

Anderson, C. L.   1936.   "Epilepsy in the state of Michigan."   *Mental Hygiene*, July, pp. 457–458.

Anspach, Renee R.   1979.   "From stigma to identity politics: political activism among the physically disabled and former mental patients."   *Social Science and Medicine* 13A:765–773.

Arluke, Arnold.   1980.   "Judging drugs: Patients' conceptions of therapeutic efficacy in the treatment of arthritis."   *Human Organization* 39:84–86.

Bagley, Christopher.   1971.   *The Social Psychology of the Epileptic Child*. London: Routledge and Kegan Paul.

Balint, Michael.   1972.   *The Doctor, His Patient, and the*

Illness. Rev. ed. New York: International Universities Press.

Becker, Howard S. 1963. *Outsiders*. New York: Free Press.

————. 1967. "Whose side are we on?" *Social Problems* 14:239–247.

————. 1973. "Labeling theory reconsidered." In *Outsiders*, pp. 177–208. New York: Free Press.

Bennett, A. E. 1965. "Mental disorders associated with temporal lobe epilepsy." *Diseases of the Nervous System* 26:275–280.

Benoliel, Jeanne Quint. 1975. "Childhood diabetes: The commonplace in living becomes uncommon." In *Chronic Illness and the Quality of Life*, ed. Anselm L. Strauss and Barney G. Glaser, pp. 89–98. St. Louis: Mosby.

Beran, Roy G., Valerie R. Jennings, and Tim Read. 1981. "Doctors' perspectives of epilepsy." *Epilepsia* 22: 397–406.

Beran, Roy G. and Tim Read. 1983. "A survey of doctors in Sydney, Australia: Perspectives and practices regarding epilepsy and those affected by it." *Epilepsia* 24: 79–104.

Bittner, Egon. 1973. "Objectivity and realism in sociology." In *Phenomenological Sociology: Issues and Applications*, ed. George Psathas, pp. 109–128. New York: Wiley.

Blaxter, Mildred. 1976. *The Meaning of Disability*. New York: Neale Watson Academe Publications, Inc.

————. 1978. "Diagnosis as category and process: The case of alcoholism." *Social Science and Medicine* 12:9–17.

Bluebond-Langner, Myra. 1978. *The Private Worlds of Dying Children*. Princeton, N.J.: Princeton University Press.

Blumer, Herbert. 1969. *Symbolic Interactionism*. Englewood Cliffs, N.J.: Prentice-Hall.

Bogdan, Robert, and Douglas Biklin. 1977. "Handicapism." *Social Policy* 7:14–19.

Bogdan, Robert, and Steven Taylor. 1982. *Inside Out: The Social Meaning of Mental Retardation.* Toronto: University of Toronto Press.

Borman, Leonard D., James Davies, and David Droge. 1980. "Self-help groups for people with epilepsy." In *A Multidisciplinary Handbook of Epilepsy*, ed. B. Hermann. Springfield, Ill.: Thomas.

Boston Women's Health Book Collective. 1973. *Our Bodies, Our Selves: A Book by and for Women.* New York: Simon and Schuster.

Burton, Lindy. 1975. *The Family Life of Sick Children.* London: Routledge and Kegan Paul.

Cannon, William B. 1932. *The Wisdom of the Body.* New York: Norton.

Caveness, William F., and George H. Gallup. 1980. "A survey of attitudes toward epilepsy in 1979 with an indication of trends over the last thirty years." *Epilepsia* 21:509–518.

Caveness, William F., H. Houston Merritt, and George H. Gallup, Jr. 1974. "A survey of public attitudes towards epilepsy in 1974 with an indication of trends over the past twenty-five years." *Epilepsia* 15: 523–536.

Center for Urban Affairs and Policy Research. Epilepsy in the Urban Environment Project. No date. *Selected Letters in Response to Advertisements Requesting Information about Non-Medical Approaches to Coping with Epilepsy.* Evanston, Ill.: Center for Urban Affairs and Policy Research, Northwestern University.

Chorover, Stephan L. 1973. "Big brother and psychotechnology." *Psychology Today*, October, pp. 43–54.

Clark, L. Pierce. 1917. "A further study of mental content in epilepsy." *Psychiatric Bulletin*, July, pp. 1–54.

————. 1925. *The Epileptic Psyche*. Stanford, Conn.: The Psychoanalytic Institute.

Clarke, Edwin. 1973. "John Hughlings Jackson." In *Dictionary of Scientific Biography*, Vol. VII, pp. 46–50. New York: Scribner's.

Comaroff, Jean, and Peter Maguire. 1981. "Ambiguity and the search for meaning: Childhood leukaemia in the modern clinical context." *Social Science and Medicine* 15B:115–123.

Commission for the Control of Epilepsy and its Consequences. 1978. *Plan for Nationwide Action on Epilepsy*. Vols. I–IV, U.S. Department of Health, Education and Welfare, pub. no. (NIH) 78-276, p. 20. (Cited as *Commission Report*.)

Conrad, Peter. 1975. "The discovery of hyperkinesis: Notes on the medicalization of deviant behavior." *Social Problems* 23 (October): 12–21.

————. 1976. *Identifying Hyperactive Children: The Medicalization of Deviant Behavior*. Lexington, Mass.: D.C. Heath.

Conrad, Peter, and Joseph W. Schneider. 1980. *Deviance and Medicalization: From Badness to Sickness*. St. Louis: Mosby.

Coombs, Robert H. 1978. *Mastering Medicine*. New York: Free Press.

Corbin, Juliet, and Anselm Strauss. 1982. "Trajectory and work and biography." Unpublished paper. Department of Social and Behavioral Sciences, School of Nursing, University of California, San Francisco.

Cowie, Bill. 1976. "The cardiac patient's perception of his heart attack." *Social Science and Medicine* 10: 87–96.

Danesi, M. A., K. A. Odusote, O. O. Roberts and E. O. Adu. 1981. "Social problems of adolescent and adult epileptics in a developing country, as seen in Lagos, Nigeria." *Epilepsia* 22:689–696.

Danziger, Sandra. 1978. "The uses of expertise in doctor-patient encounters during pregnancy." *Social Science and Medicine* 12A:359–367.

Davis, Alan, and Gordon Horobin, eds. 1977. *Medical Encounters: The Experience of Illness*. New York: St. Martin's.

Davis, Fred. 1961. "Deviance disavowal: The management of strained interaction by the visibly handicapped." *Social Problems* 9 (Fall): 120–132.

———. 1963. *Passage through Crisis*. Indianapolis: Bobbs-Merrill.

Davis, Marcella. 1973. *Living with Multiple Sclerosis*. Springfield, Ill.: Charles C. Thomas.

DeJong, Gerben. 1979. "Independent living: From social movement to analytic paradigm." *Archives of Physical Medicine and Rehabilitation* 60:435–446.

Delgado-Escueta, Antonio V., Richard Mattson, Lambert King, Eli Goldensohn, Herbert Spiegel, Jack Madsen, Paul Carandell, Fritz Dreifuss, Roger J. Porter. 1981. "The nature of aggression during epileptic seizures." *New England Journal of Medicine* 305(12): 711–716.

Deutscher, Irwin. 1973. What We Say/What We Do: Sentiments and Acts. Glencoe, Ill.: Scott, Foresman.

Dingwall, Robert. 1976. *Aspects of Illness*. New York: St. Martins.

Dohrenwend, Barbara S., and Bruce P. Dohrenwend, eds. 1974. *Stressful Life Events: Their Nature and Effects*. New York: Wiley.

Dohrenwend, Bruce P., and Barbara S. Dohrenwend. 1976. "Sex differences and psychiatric disorders." *American Journal of Sociology* 81:1447–1454.

Douglas, Mary. 1963. *Purity and Danger*. London: Routledge and Kegan Paul.

Epilepsy Foundation of America. 1976. *The Legal Rights of Persons with Epilepsy*. Washington, D.C.: Epilepsy Foundation of America.

Estes, C. L., and L. E. Gerard. 1979. "Social research in health and medicine: A selected bibliography." In *Hand-*

book of Medical Sociology, ed. H. Freeman, S. Levine, and L. Reeder, 3rd ed., pp. 475–504. Englewood Cliffs, N.J.: Prentice-Hall.

Fabrega, Horacio, Jr. 1979. "The ethnography of illness." *Social Science and Medicine* 13A:565–576.

Fagerhaugh, Shizuko. 1975. "Getting around with emphysema." In *Chronic Illness and the Quality of Life*, ed. Anselm L. Strauss and Barney G. Glaser, pp. 99–107. St. Louis: Mosby.

Featherstone, Helen. 1980. *A Difference in the Family*. New York: Penguin.

Feinstein, Abram R. 1967. *Clinical Judgment*. Baltimore: Williams and Wilkins.

Freidson, Eliot. 1960. "Client control and medical practice." *American Journal of Sociology* 65:374–382.

———. 1970. *Profession of Medicine*. New York: Dodd, Mead.

Foxe, A. 1948. *The Antisocial Aspects of Epilepsy*. London: Heinemann.

Garfinkel, Harold. 1967. *Studies in Ethnomethodology*. Englewood Cliffs, N.J.: Prentice-Hall.

Gastaut, H. 1970. "Clinical and electroencephalographical classification of epileptic seizures." *Epilepsia* 11:101.

Geist, Harold. 1962. *The Etiology of Idiopathic Epilepsy*. New York: Exposition Press.

Glaser, Barney G. 1978. *Theoretical Sensitivity*. Mill Valley, California: Sociology Press.

Glaser, Barney G., and Anselm L. Strauss. 1964. "Awareness contexts and social interaction." *American Sociological Review* 29:669.

———. 1965. *Awareness of Dying*. Chicago: Aldine.

———. 1967. ' *The Discovery of Grounded Theory*. Chicago: Aldine.

———. 1968. *Time for Dying*. Chicago: Aldine.

Goffman, Erving. 1956. "Embarrassment and social organization." *American Journal of Sociology* 62: 264–271.

———. 1959. "The moral career of the mental patient." *Psychiatry* 22:123–135.

———. 1961. *Asylums.* Garden City, New York: Doubleday.

———. 1963. *Stigma.* Englewood Cliffs, N.J.: Prentice-Hall.

Gross, M. D., and W. C. Wilson. 1964. "Behavior disorders of children with cerebral dysrhythmias." *Archives of General Psychiatry* 11:66–68.

Guerrant, John, William W. Anderson, Ames Fischer, Morton R. Weinstein, R. Mary Jaros, and Andrew Deskins. 1962. *Personality in Epilepsy.* Springfield, Ill.: Charles C. Thomas.

Gussow, Zachary, and George S. Tracey. 1968. "Status, ideology and adaption to stigmatized illness: A study of leprosy." *Human Organization* 27(4):316–325.

Harrison, T. R. 1980. *Harrison's Principles of Internal Medicine.* 9th ed. New York: McGraw-Hill.

Hauck, Vernon E. 1973. "Epilepsy and Fair Employment." Ph.D. Diss., University of Alaska, Anchorage.

Hauser, W. A., V. E. Anderson, R. B. Lowenson, and S. M. Roberts. 1982. "Seizure recurrence after a first unprovoked seizure." *New England Journal of Medicine* 307:522–528.

Hauser, W. Allen, and Leonard T. Kurland. 1975. "The epidemiology of epilepsy in Rochester, Minnesota, 1935 through 1967." *Epilepsia* 16:1–66.

Henry, Jules. 1971. *Pathways to Madness.* New York: Random House.

Hermann, Bruce P., Mark S. Schwartz, Steven Whitman and William F. Karnes. 1980. "Aggression and Epilepsy: Seizure-type comparisons and high-risk variables." *Epilepsia* 22:691–698.

―――. 1981. "Psychosis and Epilepsy: Seizure-type comparisons and high-risk variables." *Journal of Clinical Psychology* 37(4):714–721.

Hewitt, John P., and Peter M. Hall. 1973. "Social problems, problematic situations, and quasi-theories." *American Sociological Review* 38:367–374.

Hewitt, John P., and Randall Stokes. 1975. "Disclaimers." *American Sociological Review* 40:1–11.

Hicks, Robert A., and Maralee J. Hicks. 1968. "Changes over a 10-year period (1956–66) in employer's attitudes toward the employment of epileptics." *American Corrective Therapy Journal* 22:145–147.

―――. 1978. "The attitude of major companies toward the employment of epileptics: An assessment of two decades of change." *American Corrective Therapy Journal* 32:180–182.

Highmore, A. 1822. *A Treatise on The Law of Idiocy and Lunacy*. Exeter, N.H.: George Lanson and J. J. Williams.

Hopkins, Anthony, and Graham Scambler. 1977. "How doctors deal with epilepsy." *Lancet*, January, pp. 183–186.

Hughes, Everett C. 1945. "Dilemmas and contradictions of status." *American Journal of Sociology* 50:353.

―――. 1958. *Men and Their Work*. New York: Free Press.

Hughes, Kathleen. 1975. "The Person with Epilepsy in the Eyes of Society and the Law." Unpublished Senior Honors Thesis, Brandeis University.

Idler, Ellen L. 1979. "Definitions of health and illness in medical sociology." *Social Science and Medicine* 13A:723–31.

Kendall, Patricia L., and George G. Reader. 1979. "Contributions of sociology to medicine." In *Handbook of Medical Sociology*, ed. H. E. Freeman, S. Levine, and

L. G. Reeder, 3rd ed., pp. 1–22. Englewood Cliffs: Prentice-Hall.

Kitsuse, John I. 1962. "Societal reaction to deviant behavior." *Social Problems* 9:247–256.

———. 1980. "Coming out all over: Deviants and the politics of social problems." *Social Problems* 28: 1–13.

Kittrie, Nicholas N. 1971. *The Right To Be Different.* New York: Penguin.

Koos, Earl L. 1954. *The Health of Regionville.* New York: Columbia University Press.

Korsch, Barbara M., and Vida Francis Negrete. 1972. "Doctor-patient communication." *Scientific American*, August, pp. 66–74.

Korsch, B., E. Gozzi, and V. Francis. 1968. "Gaps in doctor-patient communication: Doctor-patient interaction and satisfaction." *Pediatrics* 42:855–871.

Laidlaw, John, and Alan Richens. 1976. *A Textbook of Epilepsy.* Edinburgh: Churchill Livingstone.

Lear, Martha Weinman. 1980. *Heartsounds.* New York: Simon and Schuster.

Lemert, Edwin M. 1951. *Social Pathology.* New York: McGraw-Hill.

———. 1962. "Paranoia and the dynamics of exclusion." *Sociometry* 25:7–15.

Lennox, Gordon W., and Margaret A. Lennox. 1960. *Epilepsy and Related Disorders.* Vol. I. Boston: Little, Brown.

Levine, Sol, and Martin A. Kozloff. 1978. "The sick role: Assessment and Overview." In *Annual Review of Sociology,* ed Ralph H. Turner, James Coleman, and Renee Fox, pp. 317–343. Palo Alto, Calif.: Annual Reviews, Inc.

Litman, Theodor J. 1974. "The family as a basic unit in health and medical care: A social behavioral view." *Social Science and Medicine* 8:495–519.

————. 1976. *The Sociology of Medicine and Health Care: A Research Bibliography*. San Francisco: Boyd and Fraser.

Locker, David. 1981. *Symptoms and Illness: The Cognitive Organization of Disorder*. London: Tavistock.

Lofland, John. 1971. *Analyzing Social Settings*. Belmont, California: Wadsworth.

Lorber, Judith. 1975. "Good patients and problem patients: Conformity and deviance in a general hospital." *Journal of Health and Social Behavior* 16:213.

Mannheim, Herman. 1960. *Pioneers in Criminology*. Chicago: Quadrangle.

Mark, Vernon H., and Frank R. Ervin. 1970. *Violence and the Brain*. New York: Harper and Row.

Matza, David. 1969. *Becoming Deviant*. Englewood Cliffs, N.J.: Prentice-Hall.

McKinlay, John B. 1975. "Who is really ignorant—physician or patient?" *Journal of Health and Social Behavior* 16:3–11.

Mechanic, David. 1962. "The concept of illness behavior." *Journal of Chronic Disease* 15:189–194.

————. 1968. *Medical Sociology*. New York: Free Press.

Merlis, J. K. 1970. "Proposal for an international classification of the epilepsies." *Epilepsia* 11:114

Millman, Marcia. 1976. *The Unkindest Cut*. New York: Morrow.

National Epilepsy League. 1976. Personal communication to Peter Conrad.

Newmark, Michael E., and J. Kiffen Penry. 1980. *Genetics of Epilepsy: A Review*. New York: Raven Press.

Oliver, M. J. 1980. "Epilepsy, crime and delinquency." *Sociology* 14:417–439.

Parsons, Talcott. 1951. *The Social System*. New York: Free Press.

Pillemer, Karl. 1981. "Group interaction and adaptation to a chronic condition." Paper presented at annual meeting, American Sociological Association, Toronto.

Quint, Jeanne C. 1965. "Institutionalized practices of information control." *Psychiatry* 28:119–132.

Reif, Laura. 1975. "Ulcerative colitis: Strategies for managing life." In *Chronic Illness and the Quality of Life*, ed. Anselm L. Strauss and Barney G. Glaser, pp. 81–88. St. Louis: Mosby.

Reynolds, E. H., and M. R. Trimble, eds. 1982. *Epilepsy and Psychiatry*. New York: Churchill Livingstone.

Ries, Janet K. 1977. "Public acceptance of the disease concept of alcoholism." *Journal of Health and Social Behavior* 18:338–344.

Robinson, David. 1971. *The Process of Becoming Ill*. London: Routledge and Kegan Paul.

Rodin, E. 1978. Personal Communication. Cited in *Plan for Nationwide Action on Epilepsy*, ed. Commission for the Control of Epilepsy and its Consequences, Vol. II, Pt. 1, p. 241.

Roth, Julius. 1963. *Timetables*. Indianapolis: Bobbs-Merrill.

Rothman, David J. 1971. *The Discovery of the Asylum*. Boston: Little, Brown.

Ruzek, Sheryl Burt. 1979. *The Women's Health Movement: Feminist Alternatives to Medical Control*. New York: Praeger.

Ryan, Rosemary, Ken Kempner, and Arthur C. Emlen. 1980. "The stigma of epilepsy as a self-concept." *Epilepsia* 21:433–443.

Schneider, Joseph W., and Peter Conrad. 1980. "In the closet with illness: Epilepsy, stigma potential, and information control." *Social Problems* 28:32–44.

———. 1981. "Medical and sociological typologies: The case of epilepsy." *Social Science and Medicine* 15A:211–219.

Schutz, Alfred. 1971. *Collected Papers. Volume I: The Problem of Social Reality*. The Hague: Martinus Nijhoff.

Schwartz, Raymond P. 1978. "Epilepsy employment: A historical perspective." In *Plan for Nationwide Action on Epilepsy*, ed. Commission for the Control of Epilepsy and its Consequences, Vol. II, Pt. 1, pp. 491–546.

Segall, Alexander. 1976. "The sick role concept: Understanding illness behavior." *Journal of Health and Social Behavior* 17:163–170.

Self-Help Development Institute. 1980. *Epilepsy Self-Help Workbook*. Evanston, Ill.: Self-Help Development Institute.

Skipper, James K., Jr., Daisy L. Tagliacozzo, and Hans O. Mauksch. 1964. "Some possible consequences of limited communication between patients and hospital functionaries." *Journal of Health and Human Behavior* 5:34–39.

Sofijanov, Nikola G. 1982. "Clinical Evolution and Prognosis of childhood epilepsies." *Epilepsia* 23:61–69.

Sontag, Susan. 1978. *Illness as Metaphor*. New York: Farrar, Straus and Giroux.

Speedling, Edward J. 1982. *Heart Attack: The Family Response at Home and in the Hospital*. New York: Tavistock.

Stewart, David C., and Thomas J. Sullivan. 1982. "Illness behavior and the sick role in chronic disease: The case of multiple sclerosis." *Social Science and Medicine* 16:1307–1404.

Stimson, Gerry V. 1975. "Obeying doctor's orders: A view from the other side." *Social Science and Medicine* 8:97–104.

Stimson, Gerry, and Barbara Webb. 1975. *Going to See the Doctor*. London: Routledge and Kegan Paul.

Strauss, Anselm L., and Barney G. Glaser. 1975. *Chronic Illness and the Quality of Life*. St. Louis, Mosby.

Suchman, Edward A. 1965a. "Social patterns of illness and medical care." *Journal of Health and Human Behavior* 6:2–16.

———. 1965b. "Stages of illness and medical care." *Journal of Health and Human Behavior* 6:114–128.

Suczek, Barbara, Shizuko Fagerhaugh, Anselm Strauss, and Carolyn Wiener. 1982. "Sentimental work in the technologized hospital." *Sociology of Health and Illness* 4:254–278.

Sullivan, Margaret Walker. 1981. *Living with Epilepsy*. Modesto, Calif.: Bubba Press.

Sykes, Gresham M., and David Matza. 1957. "Techniques of neutralization: a theory of delinquency." *American Sociological Review* 22:667–670.

Szasz, Thomas S. 1970. *The Manufacture of Madness*. New York: Harper and Row.

Szsaz, Thomas S., and Marc H. Hollender. 1956. "The basic models of the doctor-patient relationship." *Archives in Internal Medicine* 97:585–592.

Tagliacozzo, Daisy L., and Hans O. Mauksch. 1979. "The patient's view of the patient's role." In *Patients, Physicians, and Illness*, ed. E. Gartly Jaco, 3rd ed., pp. 185–201. New York: Free Press.

Temkin, Oswei. 1971. *The Falling Sickness*. 2nd ed. Baltimore: Johns Hopkins Press.

Thomas, David. 1982. *The Experience of Handicap*. London: Methuen.

Thurston, Jean Holowach, Don L. Thurston, Barbara B. Hixon, and Amy J. Keller. 1982. "Prognosis in childhood epilepsy." *New England Journal of Medicine* 306 (14):831–836.

Torrey, E. Fuller. 1973. *The Mind Game: Witchdoctors and Psychiatrists*. New York: Bantam.

Twaddle, Andrew C. 1981. *Sickness Behavior and the Sick Role*. Cambridge, Mass.: Schenkman.

U.S. Department of Health, Education, and Welfare—National Institute of Health. 1975. *The NINCDS Epilepsy Research Program*. Washington, D.C.: U.S. Government Printing Office.

Veith, Ilza. 1965. *Hysteria: The History of a Disease*. Chicago: University of Chicago.

Voysey, Margaret. 1975. *A Constant Burden: The Reconstruction of Family Life*. London: Routledge and Kegan Paul.

Waddell, Charles. 1982. "The process of neutralization and the uncertainties of cystic fibrosis." *Sociology of Health and Illness* 4:210–220.

Waitzkin, Howard. 1976. "Information control and the micropolitics of health care: Summary of an ongoing research project." *Social Science and Medicine* 10: 263–270.

Waitzkin, Howard B., and Barbara Waterman. 1974. *The Exploitation of Illness in Capitalist Society*. Indianapolis: Bobbs-Merrill.

Wallace, Jennifer J. 1982. "Social Support in the lives of people with a stimatizing condition: The case of epilepsy." Unpublished paper. Department of Sociology, Northwestern University, Evanston, Ill.

Watson, Lydall. 1981. *Lightning Bird*. New York: E. P. Dutton.

Wertz, Richard W., and Dorothy C. Wertz. 1977. *Lying-In: A History of Childbirth in America*. New York: Free Press.

West, Candace. 1983. "'Ask me no questions . . .': A study of queries and replies in physician-patient dialogues." In *The Social Organization of Doctor-Patient Communication*, ed. Sue Fisher and Alexandra Todd. Washington, D.C.: Center for Applied Linguistics.

West, Patrick B. 1979a. "Making sense of epilepsy." In *Research in Psychology and Medicine*, ed. D. J. Osborne, M. M. Gruneberg and J. R. Eiser, Vol. 2, pp. 162–169. New York: Academic.

————. 1979b. "An investigation into the social construction and consequences of the label epilepsy." *Sociological Review* 27:719–741.

————. 1982. "Acknowledging epilepsy: Improving professional management of stigma and its consequences." Unpublished paper. Institute of Medical Sociology.

Westburn Road, Aberdeen AB9 2ZE, Scotland.

Whitman, Steven, Bruce P. Hermann, and Andrew Gordon. 1981. "Psychopathology in epilepsy: How great is the risk?" Unpublished paper. Center for Urban Affairs and Policy Research, Northwestern University. Evanston, Ill.

Whitman, Steven, Lambert King, Tina Coleman, Cecil Patmon, Bindu Desai, and Robert Cohen. 1982. "Socioeconomic correlates of epilepsy: An epidemiological study in a U.S. prison system." Unpublished paper. Center for Urban Affairs and Policy Research, Northwestern University. Evanston, Ill.

Wiener, Carolyn L. 1975. "The burden of rheumatoid arthritis." In *Chronic Illness and the Quality of Life*, ed. Anselm L. Strauss and Barney G. Glaser, pp. 71–80. St. Louis: Mosby.

Winston, Norma. 1982. "Cancer, chemotherapy, and calendars." Unpublished paper. College of Education, Drake University, Des Moines, Iowa.

Wolfson, R. G. 1960. "Counseling the epileptic." *Vocational Guidance Quarterly* 9:35–36.

Yarrow, Marian Radke, Charlotte Green Schwartz, Harriet S. Murphy, and Leila Calhoun Deasy. 1955. "The psychological meaning of mental illness in the family." *Journal of Social Issues* 11:12–24.

Zborowski, Mark. 1952. "Cultural components in responses to pain." *Journal of Social Issues* 8:16–30.

———. 1969. *People in Pain*. San Francisco: Jossey-Bass.

Ziegler, Robert G. 1981. "Impairments of control and competence in epileptic children and families." *Epilepsia* 22:339–346.

Zola, Irving Kenneth. 1972. "Medicine as an institution of social control." *Sociological Review* 20:487–504.

———. 1973. "Pathways to the doctor—from person to patient." *Social Science and Medicine* 7:677–690.

————. 1979. "Helping one another: A speculative history of the self-help movement." *Archives of Physical Medicine and Rehabilitation* 60:452–456.

————. 1981. "Structural constraints in the doctor-patient relationship: the case of non-compliance." In *The Relevance of Social Science for Medicine*, ed. L. Eisenberg and A. Kleinman, pp. 241–252. Dordrecht: D. Reidel.

————. 1982a. *Missing Pieces: A Chronicle of Living With a Disability*. Philadelphia: Temple University Press.

————. 1982b. *Ordinary Lives: Voices of Disability and Disease*. Cambridge, Mass.: Applewood.

Index

Authors

Subjects